Contact & Occupational Dermatology

Visit our website at **www.mosby.com**

CONTACT & OCCUPATIONAL DERMATOLOGY

JAMES G. MARKS, Jr., MD

Professor and Chairman
Department of Dermatology
The Pennsylvania State University College of Medicine
The Milton S. Hershey Medical Center
Hershey, Pennsylvania

PETER ELSNER, MD

Professor and Chairman
Department of Dermatology and Allergology
Friedrich Schiller University
Jena, Germany

VINCENT A. DELEO, MD

Associate Professor of Clinical Dermatology
Department of Dermatology
College of Physicians and Surgeons of Columbia University
Chairman of Dermatology
St. Luke's–Roosevelt Hospital Center and Beth Israel Medical Center
New York, New York

THIRD EDITION

with 41 *illustrations and* 70 *color plates*

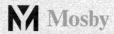

St. Louis   London   Philadelphia   Sydney   Toronto

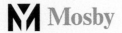

Acquiring Editor: Liz Fathman
Editorial Assistant: Paige Mosher Wilke
Project Manager: Patricia Tannian
Book Design Manager: Gail Morey Hudson
Cover Design: Teresa Breckwoldt

THIRD EDITION

Mosby, Inc.
11830 Westline Industrial Drive
St. Louis, Missouri 63146

Printed in the United States of America

International Standard Book Number 0-323-01473-9

01   02   03   04   05   TG/MV-Y   9   8   7   6   5   4   3   2   1

Preface

The purpose of the third edition of *Contact and Occupational Dermatology* remains the same as for the first and second editions. This introductory textbook is intended to be used by clinicians in their everyday practice when evaluating patients with contact and occupational dermatoses. We hope the logical approach to the patient and the "user-friendly" format presented herein are helpful in managing these patients.

We thank those individuals who used the first and second editions; we have incorporated many of their suggestions into this third edition. We have purposely not expanded the book dramatically since there are excellent encyclopedic texts on contact dermatitis that have recently been published. We think the concise and organized discussions with up-to-date information and references are sufficient for use with most patients encountered by the readers of this book.

We acknowledge those whose efforts have contributed greatly to producing this edition. Our families, again, gave us the support and time necessary to write this volume.

James G. Marks, Jr.
Peter Elsner
Vincent A. DeLeo

Introduction
How to Use This Book

Contact and Occupational Dermatology is organized for the physician to use in the diagnosis and management of suspected contact and/or occupational dermatitis. The evaluation and management of these patients require (1) a detailed history and skin examination, (2) patch testing with trays of allergens, (3) education of the patient by providing exposure lists, and (4) appropriate therapy and prevention.

The contact dermatitis patient should be scheduled for an appointment when enough time is allotted to take an extended history (Chapters 2 and 13) and when assistance is available to apply patch tests (Chapter 3). We recommend that readers photocopy the history form that is provided in Chapter 2 and use it for their patients. In addition to the history, the distribution of the dermatitis is important in directing patch testing, and Chapter 4 suggests which trays to use based on regional dermatitis distribution. In patients with suspected occupation-induced contact dermatitis, the selection of patch test trays is directed by the patient's occupation (Chapter 15).

The allergens in the text have been grouped together in Chapters 5 through 11 based on the tray in which they are found. When patch testing patients, it is helpful to think in terms of trays (e.g., Standard) rather than specific allergens (e.g., quaternium-15). With the exception of a few allergens, such as nickel, it is generally impossible to predict which specific chemical is causing the allergic contact dermatitis.

A patch test recording form is provided in Chapter 3 so that a standard format is used to document patch test reactions. Once a positive patch test result has been obtained, the exposure history is correlated with the allergen to determine relevance of the allergen to the patient's dermatitis. The relationship may not be obvious. The allergen exposure lists are helpful for the patient to pinpoint sources of the allergen that is causing the dermatitis, as well as for avoiding contact with the allergen in the future. We often review the literature concerning a particular allergen and recommend reading the section of the book that discusses the allergen.

Allergen exposure lists should be given to the patient.

Once an accurate diagnosis is made, appropriate therapy and preventive measures can be instituted (Chapters 2 and 14). Often avoidance of the irritant or allergen is curative. This, however, may not be easy (for example, in the case of a worker who may need to change professions). In other patients, the judicious use of chronic treatment, for example, topical steroids, is necessary to control the dermatitis. It must be remembered that the prognosis of occupationally induced skin disease is guarded.

We hope this text helps the reader evaluate and manage the contact dermatitis patient by integrating the history, the distribution of dermatitis, and the occupation when choosing trays of allergens for patch testing. When we have a positive patch test reaction, we read more about the allergen. We review the allergen exposure list with the patient and provide a copy of this list. For some patients, new or rare allergens may be discovered; these cases require further investigation in more encyclopedic textbooks and in journal articles.

The approach to the contact dermatitis patient should be similar to the organization of this text:
1. **Obtain a thorough history and perform a skin examination.**
2. **Patch test with trays of allergens based on history, distribution of dermatitis, and occupation.**
3. **Give allergen exposure lists to patients.**
4. **Manage with appropriate therapy and prevention.**

Contents

Contact & Occupational Dermatology

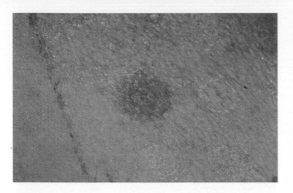

PLATE 1
Doubtful patch test reaction (?): macular erythema.

PLATE 2
Weak positive patch test reaction (+): indurated erythema.

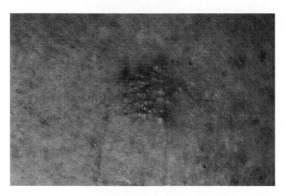

PLATE 3
Strong positive patch test reaction (++): papules and vesicles

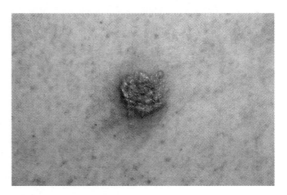

PLATE 4
Extremely strong patch test reaction (+++): confluent vesicles and bullae.

PLATE 5
Doubtful reaction (+/−) with the T.R.U.E. Test system.

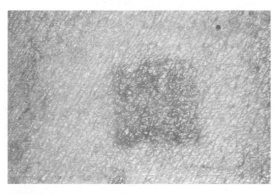

PLATE 6
A weak positive reaction (+) with the T.R.U.E. Test system.

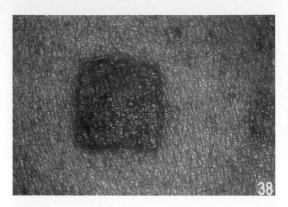

PLATE 7
A strong positive reaction (++) with the T.R.U.E. Test system.

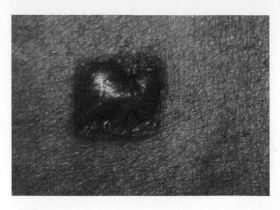

PLATE 8
An extreme bullous positive reaction (+++) with the T.R.U.E. Test system.

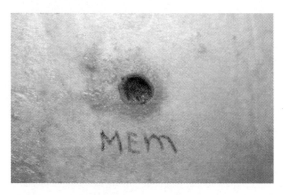

PLATE 9
Irritant reaction to monoethanolamine with necrosis of the skin and scab formation.

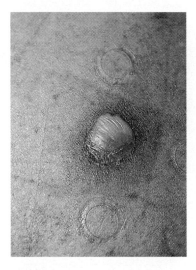

PLATE 10
An irritant pustular reaction.

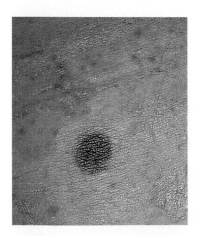

PLATE 11
An irritant response to cobalt chloride with purpura.

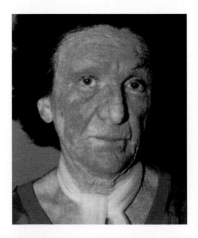

PLATE 12
Allergic contact dermatitis due to *p*-phenylenediamine found in permanent hair dye.

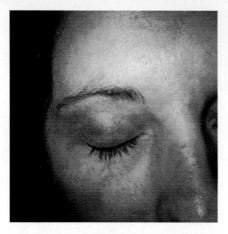

PLATE 13
Allergic contact dermatitis of the eyelid and face due to tosylamide/formaldehyde resin found in this patient's nail polish.

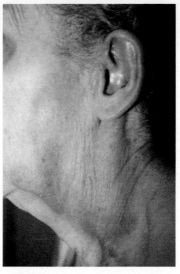

PLATE 14
Allergic contact dermatitis due to imidazolidinyl urea found in this patient's cosmetics.

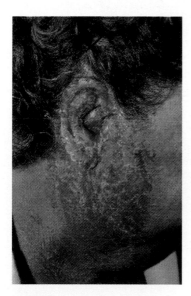

PLATE 15
Allergic contact dermatitis due to neomycin found in antibiotic eardrops.

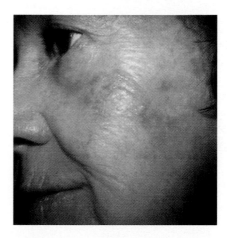

PLATE 16
A patchy facial dermatitis due to a contact allergy to thiazolinones (Kathon CG) used in moisturizer. Although the product was used extensively, the dermatitis was localized to the face and neck.

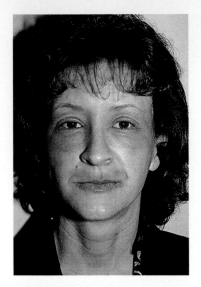

PLATE 17
Atopic dermatitis.

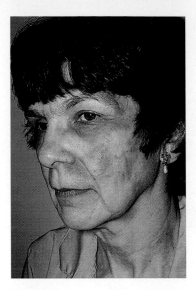

PLATE 18
Allergic contact dermatitis to poison ivy.

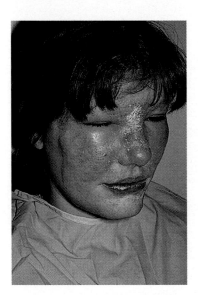

PLATE 19
Allergic contact dermatitis to poison ivy.

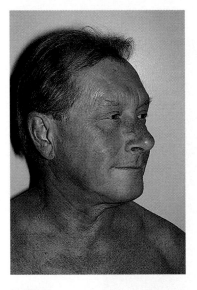

PLATE 20
Allergic dermatitis to formaldehyde-releasing preservatives in cosmetics.

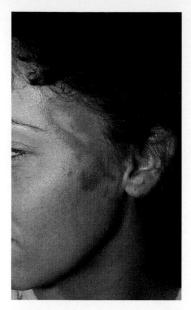

PLATE 21
Irritant contact dermatitis from a permanent wave solution.

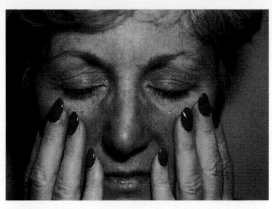

PLATE 22
Eyelid and facial allergic contact dermatitis from tosylamide/formaldehyde resin in nail polish.

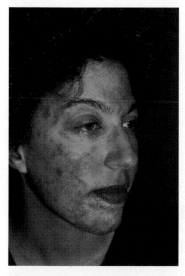

PLATE 23
Allergic contact dermatitis due to poison ivy. Note the areas of linear distribution and also the application of calamine lotion to the chin.

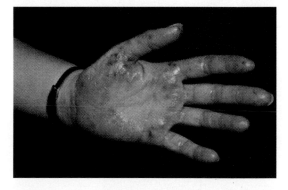

PLATE 24
This hairdresser had an allergic contact dermatitis of the hands from glycerol monothioglycolate found in permanent hair waving solution.

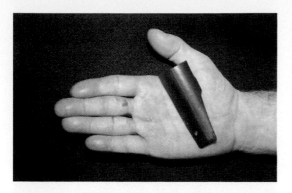

PLATE 25
This housekeeper was allergic to black rubber hoses that he handled while cleaning machinery. He had a positive patch test reaction to black rubber *p*-phenylenediamine mix (PPD mix).

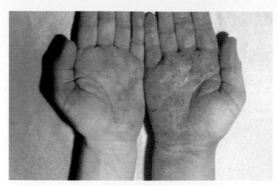

PLATE 26
This textile worker had unilateral hand dermatitis from nickel found in the scissors she used to cut fabric.

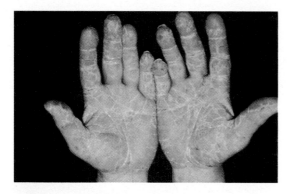

PLATE 27
This machinist had irritant contact dermatitis due to metal-working fluids. All patch test results were negative, including the metalworking fluid he used at work.

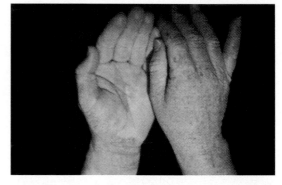

PLATE 28
This individual had allergic contact dermatitis from the rubber gloves that he wore. Patch test findings were positive to carba and thiuram mix.

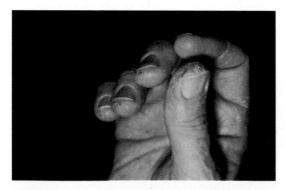

PLATE 29
This dentist was allergic to the glutaraldehyde found in the cold sterilization solutions used on his dental instruments.

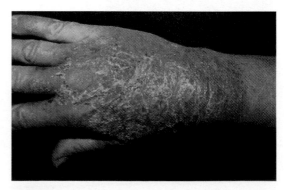

PLATE 30
This individual was allergic to benzocaine found in a medication to treat poison ivy.

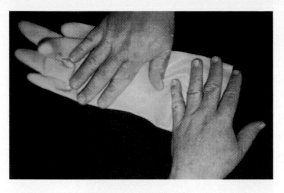

PLATE 31
This nurse was allergic to the rubber gloves she wore when taking care of patients. Patch tests revealed positive reactions to thiuram mix and a portion of her gloves.

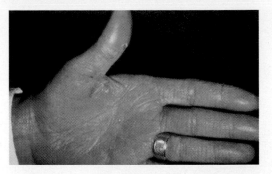

PLATE 32
This patient was allergic to quaternium-15 present in topical steroid used to treat a chronic irritant contact dermatitis. Her dermatitis flared and failed to clear when the topical steroid was used.

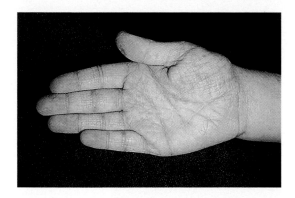

PLATE 33
Atopic dermatitis.

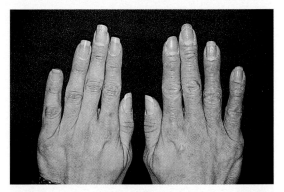

PLATE 34
Atopic dermatitis.

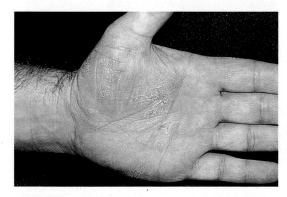

PLATE 35
Psoriasiform dermatitis.

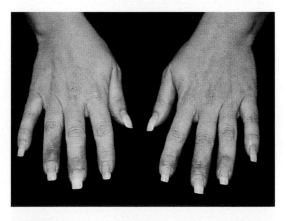

PLATE 36
Sculptured nails caused allergic contact dermatitis to the fingers.

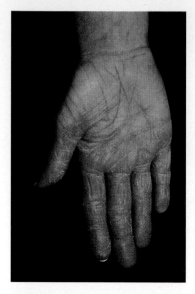

PLATE 37
Sensitivity to ethyl acrylate caused this hand dermatitis.

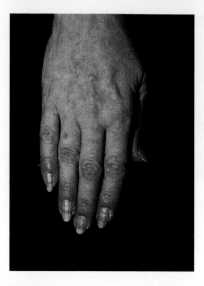

PLATE 38
Allergic contact dermatitis of the nail folds from nail polish.

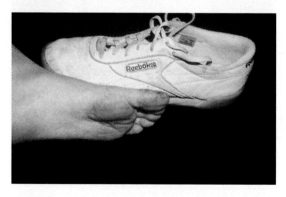

PLATE 39
This child's foot dermatitis was caused by an allergy to mercaptobenzothiazole found in her sneakers.

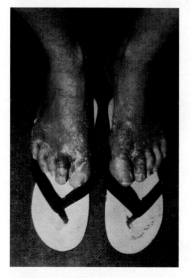

PLATE 40
This individual was allergic to mercaptobenzothiazole found in his flip-flops.

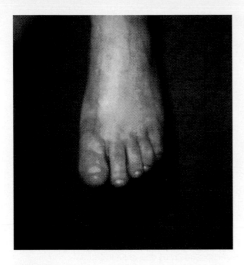

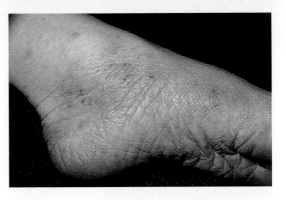

PLATE 42
Atopic dermatitis.

PLATE 41
This foot dermatitis was due to an undefined shoe component. Patch test results to parts of shoes were positive, but test responses to rubber and leather antigens in the standard and miscellaneous trays were all negative.

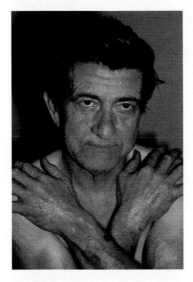

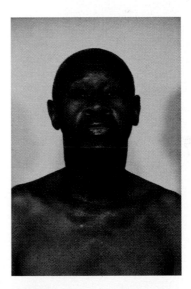

PLATE 43
Airborne allergic contact dermatitis due to black rubber from tires. He had a positive reaction to black rubber *p*-phenylenediamine mix (PPD mix).

PLATE 44
Photoallergic contact dermatitis due to musk ambrette that led to chronic actinic dermatitis. The dermatitis is limited to sun-exposed sites of the face, neck, and arms.

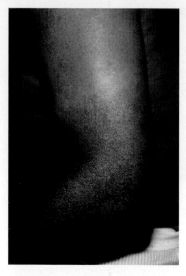

PLATE 45
Same patient as in Plate 44.

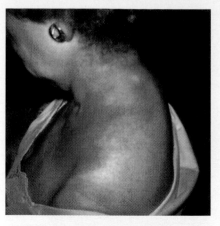

PLATE 46
Dermatitis of exposed areas due to plain contact allergy to quaternium-15 in body lotions and cosmetics. This dermatitis was *not* photoinduced or airborne in origin.

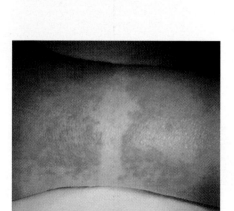

PLATE 47
Photoallergic contact dermatitis from 6-methyl-coumarin in a sun lotion. Note the sparing beneath the wristwatch.

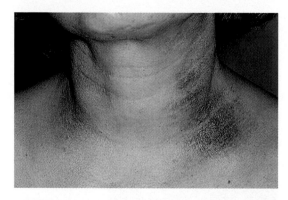

PLATE 48
Allergic contact dermatitis to tosylamide/formaldehyde resin in nail polish.

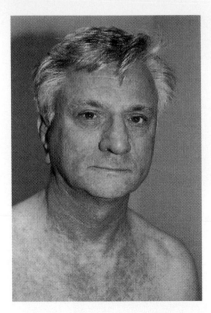

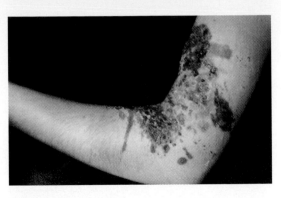

PLATE 50
This teenager was applying oven cleaner to her arm, with severe irritant contact dermatitis as a result.

PLATE 49
Allergic contact dermatitis from airborne and topical fragrances.

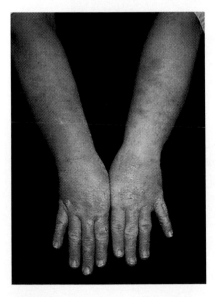

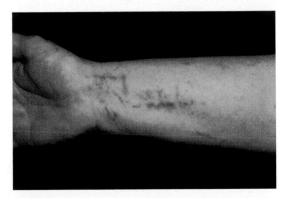

PLATE 52
Linear configuration of allergic contact dermatitis due to poison ivy.

PLATE 51
Allergic contact dermatitis from fragrance in a moisturizer.

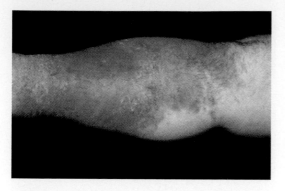

PLATE 53

This stasis dermatitis was made much worse after application of a topical antibiotic. Patch testing was positive to neomycin found in the topical antibiotic.

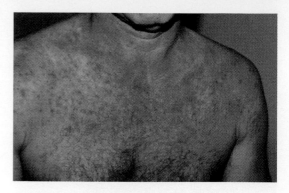

PLATE 54

Persistence of this generalized eczematous dermatitis requires patch testing to rule out an occult allergen.

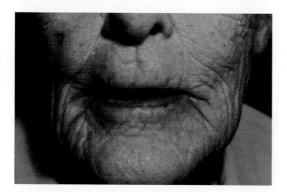

PLATE 55

Allergic contact cheilitis due to cinnamic aldehyde found in the tartar control toothpaste that this patient was using.

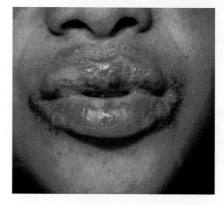

PLATE 56

Allergic contact dermatitis from oak moss, a fragrance ingredient in this patient's husband's cologne—a "consort" dermatitis.

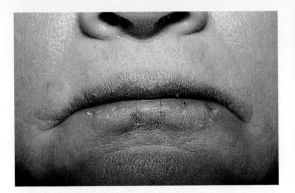

PLATE 57
Allergic contact dermatitis to Oxybenzone in lip balm.

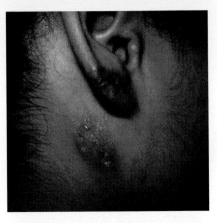

PLATE 58
Chronic allergic dermatitis due to nickel in earrings and jeans buttons. Note involvement of the earlobe and neck as well as the abdomen.

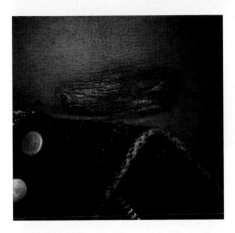

PLATE 59
Same patient as in Plate 58.

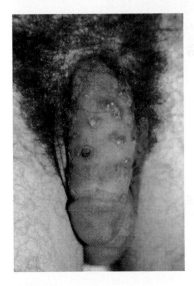

PLATE 60
Irritant contact dermatitis of the penis was induced by application of podophyllin.

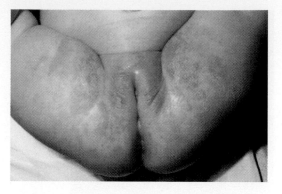

PLATE 61
Irritant contact dermatitis caused by feces and urine.

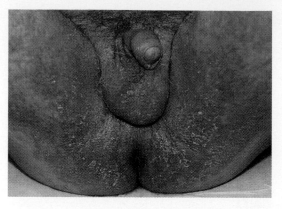

PLATE 62
This patient was sensitive to fragrance in a medicated cream.

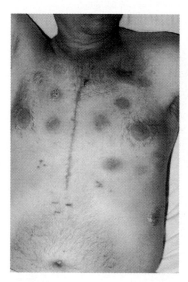

PLATE 63
Allergic contact dermatitis was produced from chloroxylenol found in electrocardiogram electrode gel.

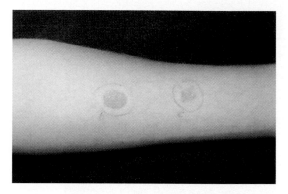

PLATE 64
Contact urticaria to benzoic acid and cinnamic acid.

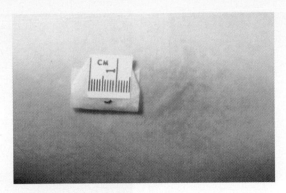

PLATE 65
Contact urticaria to a gypsy moth larva.

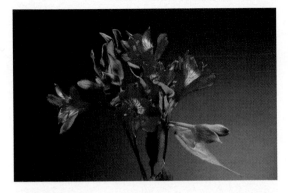

PLATE 66A
Alstroemeria.

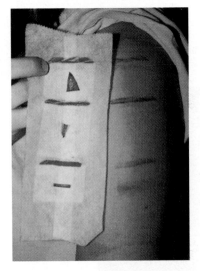

PLATE 66B
Patch test to portions of the *Alstroemeria* plant with a positive reaction to the stem.

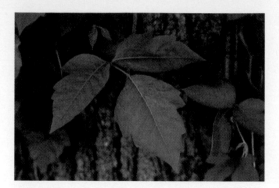

PLATE 67
Poison ivy.

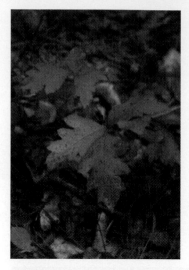

PLATE 68
Poison oak. (Courtesy of J. Guin, MD.)

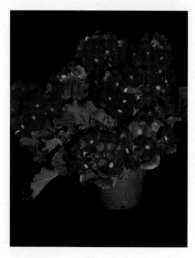

PLATE 69
Primrose *(Primula obconica).*

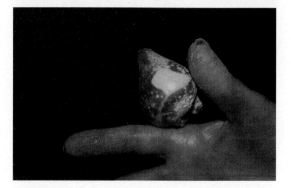

PLATE 70
Allergic contact dermatitis due to tulip bulbs, producing "tulip fingers."

PART I

Background

CHAPTER 1

Allergic and Irritant Contact Dermatitis

THE SKIN AS AN IMMUNE ORGAN
   Skin inflammation
IRRITANT CONTACT DERMATITIS
ALLERGIC CONTACT DERMATITIS
   Sensitization phase
   Elicitation phase

A number of different morphologic types of adverse cutaneous reactions may occur when skin is topically exposed to chemical agents. These diverse reactions may be due to disease or disorders produced by **contact** of the agent with any of the cells and noncellular components of the skin. The initial interaction can lead to a variety of cell- and agent-dependent biologic events resulting in a wide array of cutaneous and even systemic responses. These include localized or generalized *urticaria* with and without anaphylaxis, which is mediated by mast cell activation; *acneiform* eruptions due to changes in follicular function; alterations in melanocyte biology resulting in *hypopigmentation* or *hyperpigmentation,* interaction of the chemical agent with nonionizing radiation to induce *photosensitization* of various forms; and effects on dermal cells, supporting structures, and dermal vessels that result in *atrophy* or purpura. By far, however, the most common pathologic response pattern resulting from skin contact with a chemical agent is *eczema,* or *contact dermatitis.* **Contact dermatitis** is simply inflammation of the skin with spongiosis or intercellular edema of the epidermis that results from the interaction of a chemical and skin.

> **Diverse reactions can occur when pathologic conditions are produced in skin by contact with a chemical agent. These include urticaria, acne, hypopigmentation or hyperpigmentation, photosensitization, atrophy, purpura, and eczema.**

The response pattern of contact dermatitis is produced through one of two major pathways: **irritant** or **allergic.** Irritant contact dermatitis (ICD) and allergic

3

contact dermatitis (ACD) are two of the most common dermatologic maladies in industrialized societies, with a prevalence usually stated to be between 1% and 10%. Irritant contact dermatitis predominates and accounts for 80% of all such reactions. The number of chemical agents known to be capable of inducing ACD is said to be near 3000; the number of agents, both natural and synthetic, capable of inducing the irritant response is manyfold larger. The type of response is not totally agent specific. In fact, many highly sensitizing antigens can also be irritants, given the proper circumstances, and common irritants can also be allergens. The difference between the two responses is a very basic mechanistic one— nonimmunologic versus immunologic. Nonetheless, the more that is learned about the pathophysiology of both responses, the more similar the responses appear in many respects, including the types of cells infiltrating the skin and the soluble mediators modulating the inflammation.

Contact dermatitis
Irritant, 80%
Allergic, 20%

An allergic reaction is agent **specific,** requires sensitization, and by definition occurs only in a genetically determined segment of the population capable of being sensitized to a given antigen. Approximately 90% of the population can be sensitized to some experimental antigens like dinitrochlorobenzene, and 60% of Caucasian adults are said to be allergic to *Rhus oleoresin,* the cause of "poison ivy" dermatitis. Conversely, irritant reactions are **nonspecific** and do not require sensitization. Responses to a given irritant by definition may occur in all members of the population, but great variations in individual susceptibility to most irritants is quite common.

In clinical practice the two responses may be difficult to distinguish. Very potent irritants like hydrofluoric acid, ethylene oxide, and wet cement can result in severe skin necrosis and "chemical burns" with ulceration. Other, moderately strong irritants produce acute burning and stinging, with vesicular or bullous reactions. The vast majority of irritants in the environment, however, produce delayed or cumulative irritant reactions that become evident in the form of eczema, which is the morphologic appearance of the allergic response.

Both allergens and irritants can produce an acute eczematous picture with vesicles and weeping; subacute eczema with erythema, scaling, juicy papules, and weeping; or chronic eczema with hyperkeratosis, fissuring, and lichenification. The distinction among acute, subacute, and chronic may be chronologic and evolve from one to another. More likely, with both irritants and allergens, the morphologic appearance relates to the nature of the chemical agent, the specifics of the exposure, the general environment, and/or the responsiveness of the host (Table 1-1). As mentioned previously, many chemicals can act as both irritants and allergens. Certain agents like acids and alkalies, detergents, and solvents are by virtue of their chemical structure more likely to produce irritation. Factors related to concentration, vehicle, and duration of exposure, however, determine the irritant potential of these agents. Similarly, although the concentration of an agent is

Table 1-1	Factors Affecting Individual Cutaneous Responses to Chemical Contact
Related to the chemical 　Chemical structure 　Physical properties Related to exposure 　Concentration of the chemical 　Vehicle 　Duration of exposure 　Occlusion	Related to the individual 　Age 　Genetics 　Other skin disease or disorder 　Area of exposure Related to environment 　Humidity 　Temperature 　Wind

said to be less critical in producing an allergic response, concentration, vehicle, duration, and other factors related to the exposure, like the presence or absence of occlusion, play a role in determining whether both sensitization and elicitation of an allergic response occur.

Host factors are important in determining whether an allergic response occurs to a given chemical agent. By definition the allergic response is specific, and only certain genetically determined individuals can be sensitized to a given allergen. Genetic factors also play a role, however, in response to irritants. For example, atopic individuals with dermatitis are more susceptible to irritation, and racial differences in such susceptibility have been suggested.

Elderly and very young individuals are more likely to develop irritant responses and less likely to develop allergic ones. Certain skin sites like eyelids are more prone to respond to both irritants and allergens than are some other body sites, and both irritation and allergy are more likely to occur if the chemical agent is applied to diseased, especially eczematous, skin.

In addition to factors related to the chemical, the exposure, and the host, the environment at the time of exposure can also affect the response of an individual to an agent. High humidity and temperature predispose to both types of responses.

Factors affecting a response to chemical contact include factors related to the *chemical,* the *individual,* the *exposure,* and the *environment.*

There are clinical differences between allergic and irritant responses (Table 1-2). Low-level irritants are more likely to produce subacute or chronic dermatitis, and only very strong irritants produce vesicles. Early in the course of the dermatitis, irritants are more likely to produce burning or stinging, whereas allergens produce itching. Once the eruption becomes chronic, however, with hyperkeratosis, lichenification, and fissuring, the two types of reactions are impossible to distinguish.

On histologic examination, the differences between allergic and irritant responses are also more clear early in the response. The early irritant reaction is more

Table 1-2	Irritant Versus Allergic Contact Dermatitis: Clinical and Histologic Differences	
Feature	**Allergic**	**Irritant**
Itch	+ + + + (Early)	+ + + (Late)
Pain, burning	+ +	+ + + + (Early)
Erythema	+ + + +	+ + + +
Vesicles	+ + + +	+
Pustules	+	+ + +
Hyperkeratosis	+ +	+ + + +
Fissuring	+ +	+ + + +
Sharp demarcation	Yes	Yes
Reaction delay after contact	Days	Minutes to hours
Spongiosis	+ + + +	+ + + +
Dermal edema	+ + + +	+ + + +
Necrotic keratinocytes	+	+ + +
Ballooning degeneration	+	+ + +
Lymphocytic infiltrate	+ + + +	+ + + +
Neurotrophilic infiltrate	+	+ + +

likely to be characterized by *necrotic* keratinocytes and *ballooning* degeneration. By the time most patients are evaluated and biopsy samples finally taken, the two responses are indistinguishable with spongiosis, lymphocytic infiltrates, hyperkeratosis, crust, and scale.

The similarity of the response on both clinical and histologic examination in later stages probably occurs because the processes differ mechanistically in early phases, whereas they are similar in the later phases. This is due to infiltration by the same cells and damage by the same chemical inflammatory mediators.

The purpose of this chapter is to discuss the pathophysiology of ICD and ACD. Since this textbook is meant for clinical practice, this discussion is not extensive. We believe, however, that an understanding of basic mechanisms aids the clinician in the proper diagnosis and treatment of patients with these diseases. For more detailed discussions of pathophysiology we refer you to the articles and books listed at the end of this chapter.

Although the irritant response is more common than the allergic one, more investigative studies have focused on the latter. As we learn more about the pathophysiology of the inflammatory process in the skin as induced by chemical agents, we begin to understand both the differences and the similarities between irritant and allergic responses. We have come to realize that "immune" cells like Langerhans' cells and T cells and "immune" mediators like histamine and complement play a role in irritant-induced reactions and that many "nonimmune" inflammatory mediators like eicosanoids are active in allergic reactions.

THE SKIN AS AN IMMUNE ORGAN

The skin is composed of the cellular epidermis and the cell-poor dermis and subcutis. Within the epidermis reside the immunologically important cells, keratinocytes and Langerhans' cells. The Langerhans' cells are of bone marrow–derived, macrophage lineage. Because they are macrophages, Langerhans' cells can take up and process antigens, and because they express human leukocyte antigen DR (HLA-DR) (major histocompatibility complex [MHC] class II molecule) on their surface, they are also capable of presenting the processed antigens to and activating certain lymphocytes (CD4+ T cells). Langerhans' cells are also capable of producing soluble factors or cytokines that can affect cell function, particularly interleukin-1 (IL-1).

The keratinocyte accounts for 95% of the cells of the epidermis. It was originally thought to be immunologically inert but is now known to participate in immune regulation, particularly when stressed or activated. Although it does not routinely express HLA-DR and therefore is incapable of presenting antigen, it can express such molecules when activated. Keratinocytes are capable of producing many mediators of inflammation that allow it to modulate the movement and function of many other cell types, most important, lymphocytes (T cells), macrophages, neutrophils, mast cells, and vascular endothelial cells. These factors include IL-1 alpha and beta, IL-3, IL-6, granulocyte-macrophage colony-stimulating factor (GMCSF), epidermal-derived natural killer cell–activating factor, transforming growth factor β, and the membrane-derived eicosanoids prostaglandin (PG) E_2 and $F_{2\alpha}$ and the lipoxygenase product 12-hydroxyeicosatetraenoic acid. Keratinocytes also express on their surface other molecules that allow them to interact directly with cells. These are called intercellular adhesion molecules (ICAMs).

Although not permanent residents of normal skin, various lymphocytes from the vasculature travel from dermal vessels into the dermis and possibly into the epidermis. Such lymphocytes are classified and identified by functional differences and surface markers. The three major classes are T cells (thymus), B cells (bone marrow), and null cells. B cells function primarily in reactions mediated by antibody production. This would include three of the classic immune-mediated inflammatory responses: type I, anaphylactic; type II, cytotoxic; and type III, immune complex (Table 1-3). Type IV reactions, or delayed hypersensitivity, are mediated by T cells. In fact, T cells predominate in the lymphocyte infiltrate in most inflammatory cutaneous diseases, including ACD and ICD. There are two functionally distinct T-cell types that are identified by their expression of either one of two surface molecules, CD4 (helper T cells) or CD8 (suppressor T cells). Helper T cells are capable of interacting with cells, such as Langerhans' cells, that express MHC class II (HLA-DR) molecules. The CD4 molecule on its surface is essential for interaction with such antigen-presenting cells.

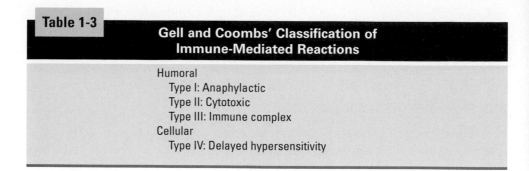

Table 1-3

Gell and Coombs' Classification of Immune-Mediated Reactions

Humoral
    Type I: Anaphylactic
    Type II: Cytotoxic
    Type III: Immune complex
Cellular
    Type IV: Delayed hypersensitivity

In addition to the CD4 molecule, antigen recognition requires another helper cell surface molecule(s). This is the α/β-peptide, heterodimer, or the *T-cell receptor/CD3 molecule complex.* The T-cell receptor is the molecule that actually recognizes or interacts with the processed antigen. The receptor is specific for the antigen. The ability of the T-cell population to be so diverse as to contain cells with receptors capable of reacting with a myriad of possible antigens is based on rearrangement of the T-cell receptor during thymic development. Such rearrangement of this receptor is the basis of the clonal theory of immune responsiveness. That is, each rearranged receptor T cell is capable of proliferating to produce a population of like cells capable of reacting to a specific antigen. The CD3 molecule is complexed to the receptor as a transduction molecule that activates the T cell on interaction with the antigen.

CD4 cells can be further subdivided into CD4 T_H1 and CD4 T_H2 cells. The cells that travel through the skin are primarily T_H1 cells. These cells differ in their production of cytokines. The profile produced by T_H1 cells include IL-2, interferon-γ (INF-γ), tumor necrosis factor β (TNF-β); that produced by T_H2 cells includes IL-4, IL-5, IL-6, and IL-10. The T_H1 cells are thought to mediate delayed hypersensitivity, whereas the T_H2 cells act to help B cells produce antibodies. The two cell types are believed to exert modulating effects on each other through their production of cytokines. INF-γ inhibits activation of T_H2 cells.

The two most well-described cytokines are IL-1 and IL-2. IL-1 is the *first signal;* it activates T helper cells. The activation includes production by the T cell of IL-2 and expression of IL-2 receptors, which leads to autocrine activation of the cell (second signal).

Besides keratinocytes, Langerhans' cells, and lymphocytes, which make up the immunologically competent skin, mast cells residing near blood vessels throughout the dermis play an important role in inflammation. Mast cells are capable of releasing histamine, various chemotactic factors, PGE_2 and PGD_2, and the leukotriene B_4 (LTB_4).

Within dermal vessels are constantly circulating neutrophils, basophils, and eosinophils awaiting the call of chemotactic factors, as well as soluble molecules like complement components and kinins able to diffuse into the dermis and epidermis whenever vascular permeability is increased.

Our understanding of the way that surface adhesion molecules participate in inflammatory reactions by allowing cells to interact with other cells has grown

Table 1-4	Cell Surface Molecules That Allow Interaction Between Cells Promoting Cutaneous Inflammation in Contact Dermatitis Reactions		
	Langerhans' Cells	T Cells	Endothelium
	ICAM-1	LFA-1	
	LFA-3	CD2	
	B$_7$	CD28	
		CLA	E-Selectin
		VLA-4	VCAM-1
		LFA-1	ICAM-1

recently. The most important of these molecules that are related to skin inflammation are listed in Table 1-4. They include ICAM-1, leukocyte function–associated antigen 3 (LFA-3), and B$_7$ on Langerhans' cells, which interact respectively with LFA-1, CD2, and CD28 expressed on T cells. Other molecules on T cells aid in the adhesion to and diapedesis through endothelium. These are CLA, very late activation (antigen) 4 (VLA-4), and LFA-1 on such cells, and their corresponding molecules are on endothelium E-selectin, vascular cell adhesion molecule 1 (VCAM-1), and ICAM-1.

Skin Inflammation

The cytokines and other soluble cell products listed earlier can either be proinflammatory or stimulatory and enhance lymphocyte activation, chemoattraction, vasodilation, and cell damage and death, or they can be antiinflammatory or regulatory and inhibit or decrease tissue damage. All of these cellular and soluble factors exist in the normal skin in a state of delicate balance. Both ACD and ICD represent a chemically induced imbalance of the stimulatory or regulatory signals responsible for immunologic homeostasis of the skin. This imbalance in ACD is triggered by exposure to a chemical (antigen) capable of reacting with specific circulating lymphocytes (primed or memory T cells), such cells having been produced in a previous sensitizing exposure to the chemical. The imbalance in ICD, by contrast, is triggered by exposure to a chemical irritant or toxin capable of directly damaging keratinocytes or possibly endothelial cells or stratum corneum. This damage results in a release of proinflammatory cytokines from the damaged cells. In either case the immune balance of the skin is upset, with resultant activation of T cells and infiltration of such cells along with neutrophils, monocytes, and other blood-borne cells into the dermis in the area of insult. This is accompanied by activation and degranulation of mast cells and vasodilation of dermal vessels. This complex cascade of events leads to the classic signs of inflammation: **redness, swelling, heat,** and **pain** (Table 1-5).

Table 1-5	Irritant Versus Allergic Contact Dermatitis: Mechanistic Differences	
Feature	**Allergic**	**Irritant**
Chemical agents	Low molecular weight, lipid soluble	Acids, alkalies, surfactants, solvents, oxidants, enzymes
Concentration of the agent	Less critical	More critical
Genetic predisposition	++++	++
Sensitization and lag period	Necessary	Not necessary
Trigger	Interaction of antigen with primed T cells	Damage to keratinocytes
Cytokine release	++++	+++
T-cell activation	Early	Later
	++++	++++
Mast-cell activation	++	++
Langerhans' cells	Increased	Decreased
Eicosanoid production	++	++

IRRITANT CONTACT DERMATITIS

By definition a cutaneous irritant is a substance that causes direct damage to skin without prior sensitization. Mechanistically, little is known about irritant contact dermatitis, but it is certain that great differences exist between the ways in which diverse chemicals damage keratinocytes. The subcellular site of such damage would be expected to vary with the chemical nature of the toxin. It is likely that the site of damage for most toxins is the lipid membrane of the keratinocyte, but some agents could diffuse through the membrane to damage lysosomes, mitochondria, or nuclear components. With membrane damage, phospholipases are activated and effect the release of arachidonic acid and the synthesis of eicosanoids (Figure 1-1). This causes activation of various second-messenger systems stimulating expression of genes, leading to the synthesis of various cell surface molecules and cytokines. Toxin treatment of skin cells has been shown to induce secretion of IL-1, which can activate T cells directly and indirectly by stimulation of GMCSF production. Eicosanoids can also affect T-cell activation and are extremely potent chemoattractants for lymphocytes as well as neutrophils. In addition, eicosanoids lead to vasodilation and increased vascular permeability directly and indirectly through mast-cell activation with histamine, eicosanoid, and platelet-activating factor production.

Infiltration by nonresident cells like neutrophils and lymphocytes into the skin at the site of toxin application, along with the diffusible factors generated by these cells and from the circulation, results in the evident clinical response to the toxin.

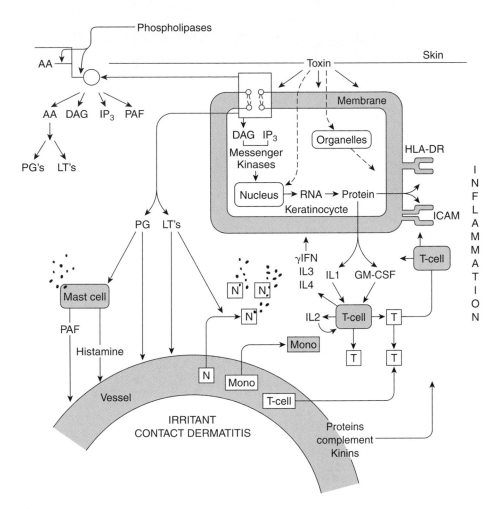

FIGURE 1-1

Irritant contact dermatitis. The chemical irritant or toxin damages the keratinocyte. This damage induces the activation of phospholipases, which release arachidonic acid *(AA)*, diacylglyceride *(DAG)*, platelet activating factor *(PAF)*, and inositides *(IP₃)*. AA is converted to prostaglandins *(PGs)* and leukotrienes *(LTs)*. Diacylglyceride and other second messengers stimulate the expression of genes and resultant synthesis of proteins. These cytokines include interleukin-1 *(IL-1)* and granulocyte-macrophage colony-stimulating factor *(GMCSF)*. IL-1 activates T helper cells to secrete IL-2 and express IL-2 receptor, which leads to autocrine stimulation and proliferation of those cells. Keratinocytes also produce the surface molecules human leukocyte antigen DR (HLA-DR) and intracellular adhesion molecule 1 (ICAM-1). PGs and LTs induce dilation of blood vessels and transudation of circulating factors of the complement and kinin systems. PGs and LTs also act as chemoattractants for neutrophils and lymphocytes and activate mast cells to release histamine and other LTs, PGs, and platelet-activating factors, thus compounding the vascular changes.

This inflammatory response is more clearly understood for a moderate irritant that produces the response on a single application. A more difficult response to define is that to a mild irritant like a detergent, which occurs only after multiple applications. In such cases the primary site of damage may be the stratum corneum, with delipidization resulting in desiccation and loss of barrier function, thus allowing for exposure of viable cells to the irritant.

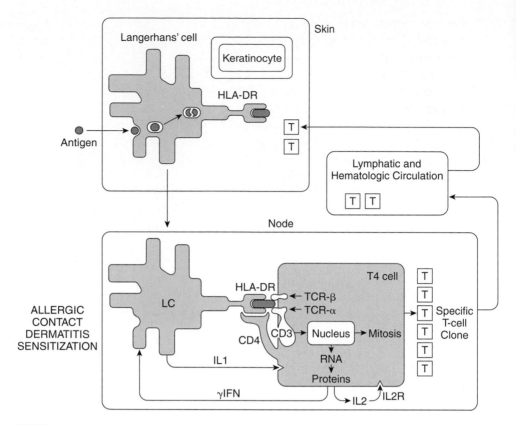

FIGURE 1-2

Allergic contact dermatitis: sensitization phase. The allergen or hapten is applied to the skin and is taken up by Langerhans' cells. The antigen is degraded or processed and bound to HLA-DR, and the complex is expressed on the surface of the Langerhans' cell. The Langerhans' cell moves via lymphatics to regional nodes, where it presents the complex to *specific CD4-positive T cells* (helper cells). The antigen–HLA-DR complex interacts with the specific T-cell receptor *(TCR)* and CD3 complex. The Langerhans' cell also secretes *IL-1*. The antigen interaction and IL-1 activate the T cell. The T cell secretes IL-2 and expresses IL-2 receptor on its surface. This causes autocrine stimulation and proliferation of specific T-cell clones (primed or memory T cells) that circulate throughout the body and back into the skin.

ALLERGIC CONTACT DERMATITIS

Allergic contact dermatitis is a classic delayed hypersensitivity, or a type IV immunologic reaction (see Table 1-3). By definition it is mediated by immune cells rather than by antibodies. The reaction can be thought of as occurring in two phases, initially a sensitization and then an elicitation response. It is the first or sensitization phase that is the basis for its classification as an immune-mediated reaction.

Sensitization Phase

The allergen is a chemical that is usually, but not always, of low molecular weight, lipid soluble, and highly reactive. An unprocessed allergen is more correctly referred to as a hapten. The hapten is applied to the stratum corneum, penetrates to the lower layers of the epidermis, and is taken up by the Langerhans' cell by pinocytosis (Figure 1-2). Within the cell lysosomal or cytosolic enzymes chemically alter the hapten, and it is conjugated to a newly synthesized HLA-DR molecule to form the complete antigen. This complex is expressed on the surface of the Langerhans' cell.

The Langerhans' cell exists in a resting or immature state and in that state functions primarily as a macrophage with little ability to stimulate T cells. When the skin is exposed to allergens, the keratinocytes secrete cytokines that produce maturation of the Langerhans' cell to an activated state, which allows them to stimulate T cells. This activation alters the phenotype of the Langerhans' cell with upregulation of secretion of certain cytokines and expression of various cell surface molecules, including Class I and II MHC, ICAM-1, LFA-3, and B_7.

The next step in the process is the presentation of the HLA-DR–antigen complex to specific helper T cells that express both a CD4 molecule that recognizes the HLA-DR of the Langerhans' cells and more specifically a T-cell receptor–CD3 complex that recognizes the processed antigen. There is some evidence that antigen can also be presented in context of the MHC class I molecules, in which case it would be recognized by CD8 cells.

The presence or absence of specific T cells is most likely genetically determined. As stated earlier, this specificity that allows interaction with thousands of antigens is developed by T-cell receptor rearrangements during early thymus development. It is unlikely that this initial HLA-DR–antigen and T-cell receptor–CD3 interaction occurs in the skin. It is believed that the Langerhans' cell migrates via the lymphatics to regional nodes where it presents the HLA-DR–antigen complex to specific T cells. Once antigen recognition occurs, both cells are activated. A series of cytokines is synthesized by both the Langerhans' cell and the T cell. Within the T cell this message is transmitted via the CD3 molecule. The Langerhans' cell secretes IL-1, which stimulates the T cell to secrete IL-2 and to express IL-2 receptors. This cytokine leads to stimulation of T-cell proliferation, thereby expanding the clone of specific T cells capable of responding to the inciting antigen. This occurs during the classic lag phase of sensitization. The primed or memory T cells that are generated are now much expanded as compared with the original population of cells with the specific T-cell receptor, and they leave the node and circulate throughout the body. The individual is now sensitized, or primed, to respond when these circulating T cells are reexposed to antigen.

Elicitation Phase

The second phase, or elicitation of the delayed type of hypersensitivity, occurs on reexposure. Once again, hapten diffuses to the Langerhans' cell, it is taken in and chemically altered, it is bound to the HLA-DR, and the complex is expressed on the surface of the Langerhans' cell. The complex interacts with primed T cells in either the skin or the node (or both), and the activation process takes place. In the skin the interaction is even more complex because other cells are present (Figure 1-3). Langerhans' cells secrete IL-1, which stimulates the T cell to produce IL-2 and express IL-2R. Once again, this leads to proliferation and expansion of the T-cell population, this time within the skin. In addition, the activated T cells secrete IFN-γ, which activates the keratinocyte and causes it to express both ICAM-1 and HLA-DR. The ICAM-1 molecule allows the keratinocyte to interact with T cells and other leukocytes that express the LFA-1 molecule. Expression of HLA-DR allows for the keratinocyte to interact directly with CD4-bearing T cells and

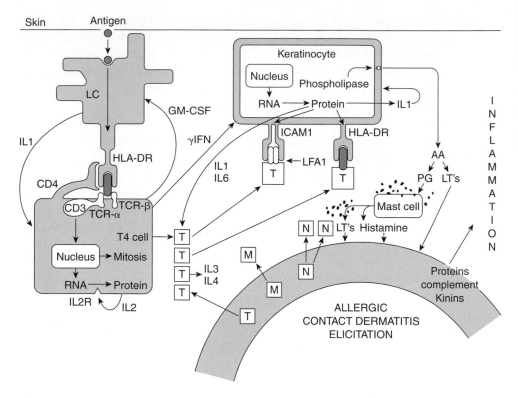

FIGURE 1-3

Allergic contact dermatitis: elicitation phase. After an individual is sensitized to an antigen, primed or memory T cells with antigen-specific TCRs are increased in number and circulate through the vasculature and into the skin. When antigen contacts the skin, it is processed and presented with HLA-DR on the surface of Langerhans' cells. The complex is presented to specific T4 cells in the skin (or node, or both), and elicitation begins. The HLA-DR–antigen complex interacts with the specific CD3-TCR complex to activate both the Langerhans' cell and the T cell. This induces secretion of IL-1 by the Langerhans' cell and results in IL-2 and IL-2R production by the T cell. This leads to proliferation of T cells. The activated T cells secrete IL-3, IL-4, IFN-γ, and GMCSF. The cytokines in turn activate the Langerhans' cell and keratinocytes. The activated keratinocytes secrete IL-1. IL-1 activates phospholipases. This releases *AA* for *PG* and *LT* production. PG and LT induce mast-cell activation and vascular dilation directly and through mast-cell histamine release. Because of the vasoactive products and chemoattractants, cells and proteins are released from the blood vessels. Activated keratinocytes also express ICAM-1 and HLA-DR, which allow for their direct cellular interaction with blood-borne cells.

may allow for antigen presentation to these cells as well. In addition, HLA-DR expression may make the keratinocyte the target for cytotoxic T cells. Activated keratinocytes also produce a number of cytokines, including IL-1, IL-6, and GMCSF, all of which can further expand the involvement and activation of T cells. In addition, IL-1 can stimulate keratinocytes to produce eicosanoids. This combination of cytokines and eicosanoids leads to activation of mast cells and macrophages. Histamine from mast cells and eicosanoids from mast cells, keratinocytes, and infiltrating leukocytes lead to vascular dilation and increased permeability to circulating proinflammatory soluble factors and cells. This cascade leads to the clinical ACD response of inflammation, cellular destruction, and reparative processes.

In addition to sensitization followed by the elicitation scenario outlined earlier, exposure to antigen may also result in activation of suppressor pathways. The net balance of sensitization and suppression resulting in disease or no disease on exposure to antigen depends on many factors. Presentation of a high concentration of antigen during the first exposure may result in the generation of specific suppressor T cells. Exposure to antigen through a site other than skin (e.g., orally or intravenously) may also result in specific suppressor-cell generation. Such responses may be due to exposure of T cells to antigen that has not been processed by Langerhans' cells. Many other poorly understood processes surely "downregulate" the immune response; for example, atopic individuals have a decreased capacity to be sensitized to common allergens. This effect probably resides within the T cell.

The balance between sensitization and suppression on exposure to antigen undoubtedly results most frequently in the latter effect; otherwise, allergic contact dermatitis would be a much more common problem. Such downregulation is certainly necessary for the survival of humans exposed frequently to a myriad of possible environmental allergens.

The preceding scenario is somewhat simplistic and based on both fact and conjecture. Certainly there are clinical and histologic differences between ICD and ACD; despite these distinctions, however, the end result of both reactions is remarkably similar in mechanism, even though they commence with very different triggering processes.

BIBLIOGRAPHY

Anderson KE, Benezra C, Burrows D et al: Contact dermatitis: a review, *Contact Dermatitis* 16:55-78, 1987.

Baadsgaad O, Wang T: Immune regulation in allergic and irritant skin reactions, *Int J Dermatol* 30:161-172, 1991.

Belsito DV: Pathophysiology of allergic contact dermatitis. In Soter NA, Baden HP, editors: *Pathophysiology of skin disease,* ed 2, New York, 1991, McGraw-Hill.

Cruz PD Jr: What accounts for contact allergy? *Am J Contact Dermat* 5:189-193, 1994.

Gaspari AA: Immunology of contact dermatitis, *Immunol Allergy Clin North Am* 17(3):377-405, 1997.

Jackson EM, Goldmen R, editors: *Irritant contact dermatitis,* New York, 1990, Marcel Dekker.

Rietschel RL, Fowler JF: *Fisher's contact dermatitis,* ed 4, Philadelphia, 1995, Lea & Febiger.

CHAPTER 2

Evaluation and Treatment of Patients With Contact Dermatitis

This chapter and the next deal with the diagnosis and treatment of the patient with allergic contact dermatitis. Central to that process, of course, is patch testing. Diagnosis of allergic contact dermatitis can be confirmed only by such testing. Without identification of the etiologic allergen by patch testing and subsequent instruction in allergen avoidance, treatment of the patient with allergic contact dermatitis is doomed to fail.

The process of evaluation is divided into two sections. This chapter deals with **whom** to patch test; Chapters 3 and 4 deal with the **what, when,** and **where** of patch testing.

WHOM TO PATCH TEST

The higher the level of suspicion for allergic contact dermatitis by a given clinician, the more frequently the diagnosis of allergic contact dermatitis will be made

Table 2-1	Morphologic Appearance of Disease Warranting Patch Testing
Dermatitis	Burning and itching skin with no visible disease or disorder
Erythroderma	Photosensitivity
Urticaria	Dermal inflammatory reactions

Table 2-2	Presentation of Patients With Allergic Contact Dermatitis: Whom to Patch Test

Specific antigen or substance suspected
Highly suggestive history or distribution
"Other" dermatidites that flare or do not respond to treatment
   Highly suspected
      Atopic eczema
      Stasis dermatitis
      Hand dermatitis
         Irritant contact dermatitis
         Dyshidrotic eczema or pompholyx
         Pustulosis palmaris et plantaris or psoriasis limited to the palms and soles
   Less likely
      Seborrheic dermatitis
      Chronic tinea pedis or manus
      Nummular eczema
Occupationally related dermatitis
Undiagnosed cutaneous problems and erythroderma
Special situations
   Urticaria
   Photosensitivity
   Systemic contact dermatitis

by that clinician. Any patient who seeks medical attention for a dermatitis or eczema is a possible candidate for patch testing. In addition, one must also consider contact allergy in patients with erythroderma, dermal inflammatory reactions, photosensitivity, urticarial responses, and symptoms of burning and itching skin (Table 2-1).

> In a particular clinic the *incidence* of allergic contact dermatitis is determined by the *interest* the dermatologist takes in allergic contact dermatitis.
>
> **Hjorth and Fregat**

Presentation of patients with allergic contact dermatitis may occur in one of the ways listed in Table 2-2 and discussed below.

Specific Antigen

The obvious candidate for patch testing is the individual who has a chief complaint of "allergy" to a specific substance. The most common clinical situation of this type would probably be the patient with poison ivy dermatitis; that is the one case in which patch testing is not recommended. Since allergy to poison ivy, oak, and sumac is almost universal, patch testing is not discriminating. In fact, testing to these antigens may actually induce sensitization.

Two frequent presentations are patients complaining of allergy to jewelry and to cosmetics. These patients may be incorrect in their diagnosis and may in fact have disease unrelated to cosmetics or jewelry. Even the best clinician can also be mistaken. Patch testing should usually be carried out for confirmation of the diagnosis of allergic contact dermatitis; otherwise, education in avoidance of the allergen may be difficult. With multiingredient cosmetics or other products, patch testing is, of course, essential for identification of the allergenic component.

Suggestive History or Distribution

Patients may seek medical attention with a dermatitis whose origin is unsuspected by them. The distribution, however, is strongly suggestive of contact dermatitis. Eyelid dermatitis due to nail cosmetics is a classic example. Chapter 4 presents distributions of dermatitis that should alert the clinician to consider the possibility of allergic contact dermatitis.

In some individuals the history is suggestive of contact dermatitis even if unsuspected by the patient. The inability of the patient to recognize an obvious relationship between contact and disease is usually based on widely held misconceptions about allergic contact dermatitis. Such misconceptions may also be held by physicians and even trained allergists and dermatologists (Tables 2-3 and 2-4). Probably the most common of these misconceptions relates to the timing of the allergic response. Allergic contact dermatitis routinely develops 24 to 48 hours after exposure. It may develop as early as 6 hours or as late as 7 days after exposure, but unless it is contact urticaria, it will not develop within minutes or a few hours. Most nonphysicians and even some physicians fail to recognize the delay. A recurrent dermatitis that routinely develops on Monday is not likely to be due to contact with an allergen at work but in fact is related to recurrent recreational exposure on weekends.

Another common misconception is that allergy does not occur to substances with which the patient has had long-term exposure. It is true that the offending allergen is more likely to be something of more recent exposure (a week to months). It is possible, however, to develop an allergy to agents after years of contact. It should also be remembered that components of products may be changed by manufacturers without alteration of the trade name of the product.

Patients frequently disallow as a problem, when giving a history, substances to which they have very little exposure because they believe that allergic reactions are dose dependent: "It can't be my makeup, I only wear a little of it on weekends!" or "I've only used sunscreen three or four times in the last month." Frequently exposure to sources of antigens such as eyelash curlers, steering wheels, makeup sponges (rather than the makeup itself), and writing instruments, may even escape the attention of well-trained physicians. A related fallacy is the belief that inexpensive products cause more problems than expensive products do. This

Table 2-3	Commonly Held Misconceptions About Allergic Contact Dermatitis That Alter the Patient's Ability to Recognize Offending Allergens

Fallacy: Rash quickly follows contact.
Truth: The rash is almost always delayed by 1 or 2 days and may not even appear for a week after contact.
Fallacy: Allergy develops only to new substances.
Truth: Allergy can develop after years of contact.
Fallacy: Allergy is dose dependent.
Truth: Allergy is not, within a wide range, dose dependent.
Fallacy: If change in consumer product exposure does not lead to clearing of the rash, that product is not etiologic.
Truth: Many products contain the same or cross-reacting antigens; also the composition of products may be altered without a change in trade name of product.
Fallacy: Contact allergy always occurs only at the site of exposure to the offending agent.
Truth: The dermatitis is usually most severe at the site of exposure, but because allergens may be carried to other sites, dermatitis may be more widespread; because body sites differ in responsiveness to allergens, the most severe dermatitis may occur at a site distant from the primary exposure site.
Fallacy: Negative scratch testing or a negative radioallergoabsorbent test (RAST) rules out allergic contact dermatitis.
Truth: Only patch testing is diagnostic of allergic contact dermatitis.
Fallacy: Expensive products are not allergenic.
Truth: Allergy is not cost dependent.

Table 2-4	Commonly Held Misconceptions About Allergic Contact Dermatitis That Alter the Physician's Ability to Recognize Contact Dermatitis

Fallacies

Allergic contact dermatitis is always bilateral if antigen exposure is bilateral (e.g., shoe or glove allergy).
Allergic contact dermatitis is not patchy (i.e., it is the same intensity at all areas of exposure).
Allergic contact dermatitis does not affect the palms and soles.

is probably based on a misunderstanding that allergenicity is related to toxins or infective agents in "cheap" products.

A most confusing situation relates primarily to cosmetic and personal care products like skin and body lotions. For example, an individual suspects, probably correctly, that a reaction is developing to a specific cosmetic, so she changes to a different brand of cosmetic once or multiple times. When the eruption fails to clear, the individual assumes that the cosmetics are not causative. The fallacy here is, of course, based on the belief that such products have exclusive components, when in fact they share common chemicals that may be allergenic. Similarly, patients may fail to suspect prescription or over-the-counter topical medications as problematic. This is a particularly compounding problem in the individual who has a contact allergy to medication that complicates an underlying "other" dermatitis like atopic eczema.

The distribution of an allergic contact dermatitis is usually the single most important clue to the diagnosis of the disease, and usually the area of greatest disease is the area of greatest contact with the offending allergen. Occasionally this rule does not hold, and to the patient or the untrained physician the distribution can actually lead to confusion in suspecting an allergy. The classic example is, of course, eyelid dermatitis due to nail cosmetics. Cases in which the most severe dermatitis appears in an area distant from the apparent site of contact are due to one of two factors. The first is transfer of antigen to distant sites. This is particularly common with antigens that are transferred unknowingly to other body sites by the hands, which are the only recognized site of exposure. Volatile antigens can also be transferred via air currents to exposed areas of the face and neck (airborne distribution). Second, there are intrinsic differences in the susceptibility of different body sites to respond to allergens. Facial skin, particularly eyelids, and genital skin are two areas of high reactivity. Allergy to nail polish frequently results in dermatitis of the eyelids with sparing of the hands. Eyelids may also be primarily involved in reactions to hair dye allergens, whereas scalp skin may be spared. Recently individuals with eyelid dermatitis have been found to be patch test–positive to gold. This appears to be a relevant allergen, since removal of all gold jewelry for 6 to 8 weeks results in resolution of the dermatitis. Certain areas tend to have higher or lower levels of exposure to antigens for not clearly recognized reasons. Deodorant allergy may spare the center of the axillary vault and appear on the periphery because the allergen is being "washed" by perspiration to the more distal skin areas. Allergens in moisturizing products that are used on many body areas may produce reactions predominantly in skin folds and intertriginous areas where the antigens tend to "well up" or concentrate.

Patients are unlikely to recognize the differences between humoral and cellular immune reactions. Frequently they inform the dermatologist that they have had extensive scratch testing or a blood test (radioallergoabsorbent test [RAST]) by an allergist and that the results were negative. Therefore they assume that they are not allergic. A careful but brief discussion of the differences between patch and scratch testing is usually sufficient to make patients aware of the allergic possibilities. A converse situation can also exist when an individual wrongly assumes that a positive scratch test result or RAST test reaction to an antigen like wool or dog dander means that his or her dermatitis is therefore due to that allergen. Once again, a brief but thorough discussion is necessary to develop an informed patient who is able to assist in the diagnosis and care of his or her disease.

Other Disease

Less obvious patients in need of patch testing are individuals suspected of or diagnosed as having a different cutaneous disease. These include patients who seek help initially for or who are being followed up long-term for atopic eczema; irritant contact dermatitis, especially hand dermatitis; dyshidrotic eczema or pompholyx; stasis dermatitis; pustulosis palmaris et plantaris or psoriasis limited to the hands and/or feet; seborrheic dermatitis outside of hairy areas; chronic fungal infections of the hands and/or feet; and nummular dermatitis (see Table 2-2).

When patients with a history and morphologic appearance suggestive of the preceding diagnoses first seek help from the clinician, allergic contact dermatitis should be in the differential diagnosis, but patch testing is usually not indicated because that diagnosis is somewhat low on the differential list. If, however, the patient fails to respond with improvement and clearing after adequate treatment, suspicion of allergic contact dermatitis masquerading as some "other dermatitis" should be considered, and patch testing should be performed. It should be remembered that potent topical or systemic corticosteroids may suppress allergic contact dermatitis, despite persistent allergen exposure. Flaring always occurs, however, after cessation of therapy.

An alternative situation is one in which patients are treated and cleared with confirmation of the "other dermatitis" diagnosis. Allergic contact dermatitis should be considered when an unexplained flare or worsening of disease occurs. In the latter case allergic contact dermatitis has developed and is complicating the primary disease. In many such cases the allergy is to an antigen receiving heightened exposure through damaged skin caused by the primary disease. The allergen is usually present in the topical agents, prescription or otherwise, being used to treat the primary disease.

Atopic Eczema

A great deal has been written concerning the relationship between atopy and contact dermatitis. No consensus exists concerning the relationship because the data reported are often contradictory. There has been a perception that atopic individuals should not develop allergic contact dermatitis as frequently as normal ones. This is based on in vitro studies that reveal that atopic individuals tend to mount T_H2 predominant response to allergens, whereas allergic contact dermatitis is a T_H1 mediated response. This shift in response pattern to allergen likely leads to what has been observed in in vivo studies that reveal atopics to be less easily sensitized than controls to universal antigens like poison ivy extract or dinitrochlorobenzene. This alteration in T-cell function may be primary or secondary, since it has been related to the level of activity of the atopic disease, especially dermatitis. On the other hand, clinical studies have shown rates of contact allergy in atopic study groups that are lower than, the same as, or higher than those in control groups. In addition, the reported percentage of atopic individuals in populations of patients with positive patch test results have varied: lower than, the same as, or higher than in the general population. If in fact there is more contact allergy in atopics, there is an apparent discrepancy between a deficiency in immune function and clinical disease in atopics. This is probably due to the enhancement of sensitization to allergens presented through skin with decreased barrier function. That is, atopic individuals have a baseline of decreased ability to develop sensitization because of a defect in T-cell function, but this is associated with an increased exposure at the T-cell level to processed antigen. The net effect would be that atopics are at least as likely to develop allergic contact dermatitis as normal individuals. Therefore one would expect atopics to develop more contact allergy to agents like topical antibacterials and preservatives in topical medications and emollients. In fact, increased neomycin sensitivity has been reported in atopics.

> **Atopics exhibit a decreased T-cell response to antigens but an increased exposure because of the loss of barrier function in their dermatitis-involved skin.**

On the other hand, atopics are more likely to develop irritant contact dermatitis, especially hand dermatitis from job-related exposure. This has been ascribed to an increased transepidermal water loss and a decreased ability of the skin to bind water. In fact, many clinicians consider irritant hand dermatitis in an adult as an expression of the atopic phenotype.

> **Atopics with eczema are probably at least as likely to develop allergic contact dermatitis as nonatopic individuals and more likely to develop irritant contact dermatitis.**

The atopic state may also have an effect on the interpretation of patch testing results. Atopics are more likely to develop dermal reactions with little epidermal change to some antigens. They may develop false-positive, pustular reactions to other antigens, particularly to nickel. Patch testing an individual with active eczema may also yield an "excited skin" or "angry back," leading to false-positive readings.

Stasis Dermatitis

Allergic contact dermatitis is a frequent complicating factor in the management of a patient with stasis dermatitis, especially if the patient has had frank ulcerations. The incidence of allergic contact dermatitis in patients with stasis dermatitis may in fact be higher than 50%. The offending allergen is usually a component of a medication used to treat the dermatitis, and the high level of sensitivity to such antigens is due to the decrease in barrier function of dermatitic or ulcerated skin. A high index of suspicion should always be present when treating such patients.

> **Greater than 50% of patients with stasis dermatitis, especially with ulcers, may develop allergic contact dermatitis.**

Hand Dermatitis

All patients with **chronic** hand dermatitis or hand and foot dermatitis should be patch tested, regardless of whether the diagnosis is dyshidrosis, irritant or atopic dermatitis, or pustulosis palmaris et plantaris. When to patch test such individuals must depend on the clinical setting. Whenever the dermatitis becomes intractable or if the dermatitis responds to treatment but flares immediately on cessation of topical or systemic corticosteroids, contact allergy should be suspected. It should also be remembered that the presence of foot as well as hand involvement does not rule out contact allergy. There are many antigens such as rubber components (in household gloves and rubber adhesives in shoes) to which both areas of the body share exposure.

Table 2-5	Irritant Contact Dermatitis Diagnostic Criteria

Subjective major criteria
  Onset of symptoms within minutes or hours of exposure.
  Pain, burning, stinging, or discomfort exceeding itching, especially early in the clinical course.
Subjective minor criteria
  Onset of dermatitis within 2 weeks of environmental exposure. (This is often a difficult history to elicit except in special settings where the irritant is a relatively novel rather than ubiquitous substance.)
  Many people in the environment similarly affected. (If this information is based solely on the history provided by the patient, its validity is suspect unless verified by an examining physician.)
Objective major criteria
  Macular erythema, hyperkeratosis, or fissuring predominating over vesicular change. (Vesicles may be present in irritant reactions with strong irritants, especially on the palms. When vesicles predominate, the likelihood of allergy increases.)
  Glazed, parched, or scalded appearance of the epidermis.
  The healing process proceeds without plateau upon withdrawal of exposure to the substance in question. (If not, strongly consider endogenous disease such as atopic dermatitis or psoriasis.)
  Patch testing with known environmentally relevant allergens is negative.
Objective minor criteria
  Sharp circumscription of the dermatitis.
  Evidence of gravitational influence such as a dripping effect.
  Lack of a tendency for spread of the dermatitis. (This can be properly evaluated only on sequential examinations.)
  Vesicles closely juxtaposed to patches of erythema, erosions, bullae, or other morphologic changes which suggest that small differences in concentration or contact time produce large differences in skin damage.

From Rietschel R. In Jackson EM, Goldman R, editors: *Irritant contact dermatitis,* New York, 1990, Marcel Dekker.

One of the most difficult clinical distinctions is between irritant and allergic contact dermatitis of the hands (and feet). Patch testing should be performed in all chronic cases.

One of the most difficult clinical distinctions to make is between irritant and allergic contact dermatitis of the hands. Patch testing except in very mild, transient cases is almost always indicated. Diagnostic assistance can be gained from the criteria established by Rietschel (1990) and outlined in Table 2-5. This distinction is based on both historical grounds and physical examination. While helpful, it does not usually obviate the need for patch testing.

Seborrheic Dermatitis

There are patients suspected of having seborrheic dermatitis, especially of the face, who actually have contact dermatitis. This can be particularly confusing when the dermatitis is a patchy facial dermatitis. There may be discrete subacute or chronic eczematous patches and plaques in a patient who is reacting to an antigen being applied to the entire face. A classic example of this is the photocontact allergic reaction to musk ambrette in men's aftershaves.

Tinea Pedis and Tinea Manus

Patients are frequently treated for fungal infections of the hands and feet, despite negative results of potassium hydroxide examinations or cultures. Once again, in such patients who fail to respond, allergic contact dermatitis must be considered. In addition, as with the other diseases listed in Table 2-2, contact allergy, especially to medications, can complicate the treatment of tinea pedis or tinea manus.

Nummular Eczema

Any patients with generalized, although patchy, dermatitis like nummular eczema should be considered possible candidates for patch testing if they fail to respond to therapy. The most likely antigens would be in topical medications and fabric finishes or dyes.

Occupational Disease

Occupational dermatitis is discussed extensively in another section of this book. It should be remembered, however, that most of us have "jobs" or do occupational activity, so in a general sense, an occupational history is a part of the workup of almost all patients with dermatitis.

Undiagnosed Cutaneous Problems and Erythroderma

There are patients who have a variety of histories and morphologic skin changes in whom no diagnosis is apparent, even after extensive workup and long-term follow-up. They are frequently seen by numerous physicians. Skin biopsy specimens may reveal a spongiotic dermatitis or may be less specific. The condition of such patients may be classified under a myriad of terms, including essential pruritus, xerotic eczema, possible drug eruption, neurodermatitis, and adult atopic eczema. Such patients should be patch tested. The risks of side effects, expenditure of time, and expense are warranted to rule out a possible, easily curable problem like allergic contact dermatitis. Even the most extensive directed history may fail to reveal a possible contact allergen.

The patient with *erythroderma* in whom a diagnosis of psoriasis, cutaneous T-cell lymphoma (CTCL), or drug eruption cannot be confirmed should be patch tested. It should be remembered that such patients who are in fact suffering from a generalized contact dermatitis may be found on skin biopsy to have infiltrating atypical cells in the dermis and epidermis. Such individuals may be labeled as having a suggestion of or even definite lymphoma (CTCL or mycosis fungoides). These individuals have been diagnosed as having **lymphomatoid contact dermatitis** or, in the case of photo-induced reactions, **actinic reticuloid.** Only with an extremely high index of suspicion will the correct diagnosis be made in such patients. Failure to suspect the diagnosis in these patients can cause a particularly dangerous therapeutic course. Patch testing such individuals is also extremely difficult. It may be best to hospitalize such patients to clear the disease with topical corticosteroids so that testing can be performed.

Special Situations

There are special situations that suggest to the physician that a patient should be patch tested. All patients who complain of photosensitivity or who have a photo-distributed eruption should be photo–patch tested (see Chapter 9). Patients who have urticaria or more generalized immediate types of reactions (e.g., angioedema or anaphylaxis) should be considered for a contact urticaria workup if the history is suggestive of a contact exposure as etiologic. The reaction would, of course, usually follow within minutes of exposure (see Chapter 16).

One patient who may be a candidate for patch testing is the patient who has dermatitis after systemic exposure to a chemical, usually a medication. This **systemic contact dermatitis** is presumed to be due to a delayed T-cell–mediated reaction to an agent or chemically related agent previously causing an allergic contact dermatitis. The dermatitis may be limited to areas of previous topical exposure or may be generalized. These types of cross-reactions between topical and systemic agents are discussed with the specific antigens. For example, patients sensitized to ethylenediamine may have reactions to aminophylline (theophylline plus ethylenediamine).

TAKING THE HISTORY

The initial history of a patient who will ultimately be evaluated for allergic contact dermatitis is the standard dermatologic history. At some point when contact allergy becomes suspected, the history naturally shifts to more carefully investigate exposure to possible antigens. If the patient initially complains of a reaction to a specific agent, the shift is an early one. The more educated the clinician becomes, the earlier he or she is likely to recognize the possibility of contact allergy and the more directed the history taking becomes. Frequently this shift occurs only after the physical examination and finding of a well-demarcated dermatitis.

> **If allergic contact dermatitis is suspected, schedule enough time for a detailed history and complete skin examination.**

We have included a patch test and occupational history and physical examination form for your use (Figure 2-1). While we *strongly urge use of this form* if occupational disease is suspected, an abbreviated form that concentrates on pages 1, 2, 4, and 5 will suffice for the workup of the patient with nonoccupationally related contact dermatitis.

The history begins with a discussion of the present illness and focuses on the site of onset of the problem and the topical agents used to treat the problem. A past history of skin disease, atopy, and general health is routinely investigated. This is followed by a detailed history of the usage of personal care products and cosmetics for skin, hair, and nails. The occupation should be ascertained; if that occupation appears causative, the occupational history can be taken.

Patients may inadvertently give an inadequate history because they feel that some points are of no concern. Patients may even be hostile when the possibility of a contact allergy is suggested to them. This is because they may hold one or more of the misconceptions about contact allergy as outlined in Table 2-3. Taking time to educate them as to the fallacy of their beliefs allows them to assist the clinician in the detection of possible allergens.

Text continued on p. 31

PATCH TEST AND OCCUPATIONAL HISTORY AND PHYSICAL EXAMINATION

Date: _____

Age _____ Sex M _____ F _____ Home phone _____ Work _____

Referred by (name, address) _____

_____ Phone_____

PRESENT ILLNESS

Date of onset of rash _____Site of onset _____

Patient's description of dermatitis—symptoms _____

_____

_____

_____

_____

Materials contacted <u>other</u> than at work (clothing, cosmetics, plants, chemicals, etc.) _____

_____

Present dermatologic medications _____

_____

Previous treatment at plant dispensary _____

_____

Previous treatment by physician _____

_____

_____

Previous self-treatment _____

_____

_____

Protective clothing No _____ Yes _____ Type gloves _____

_____

(Physician's signature)

FIGURE 2-1
Five-part patch test and occupational history and physical examination form (page 1). An abbreviated form, concentrating on information requested on pages 1, 2, 4, and 5, suffices for the workup of the patient with nonoccupationally related contact dermatitis.   *Continued*

PATCH TEST AND OCCUPATIONAL HISTORY AND PHYSICAL EXAMINATION

PAST HISTORY

Previous skin diseases? No _____ Yes _____ Types _____

_____

Were previous skin diseases related to occupation? No _____ Yes _____

Past health _____

_____

_____

Current nondermatologic medications _____

_____

_____

_____

Allergic history (circle and describe)

Hay fever	Asthma	Eczema	Cosmetics	Medications
Sunscreens	Jewelry	Drugs, etc. _____		

_____

Family history of asthma, hay fever, eczema? No _____ Yes _____

Hobbies _____

Sports _____

Personal habits

    Handwashing—frequency, type of soap _____

    Bathing—frequency, type of soap _____ _____

    Body lotion _____

    Hand lotion _____

    Facial makeup _____

        Base _____

        Blush _____

        Eye products _____ Eyelash curler? Yes _____ No _____

        Lipstick _____

    Deodorant _____

    Cologne, perfume _____

    Shaving cream _____

    Hair dye, bleach, etc. _____

    Laundry—frequency, type of detergent _____

    Nail cosmetics, wraps _____

    Toothpaste _____

    Contact lenses? No _____ Yes _____ Solutions _____

FIGURE 2-1, cont'd

Page 2 of five-part patch test and occupational history and physical examination form.   *Continued*

PATCH TEST AND OCCUPATIONAL HISTORY AND PHYSICAL EXAMINATION

OCCUPATIONAL HISTORY

Do you think the present dermatitis is occupationally induced?

No _____ (if no, go on to next page) Yes _____ Uncertain _____

List present and previous occupations and give dates of employment _____

_____

_____

_____

_____

Current employer (name, address) _____

_____ (Dates employed) _____

Supervisor (name) _____ Phone _____

Employer at onset of dermatitis—Same as current employer? No _____ Yes _____

If No (name and address, dates employed) _____

Job title at onset of rash _____Dates of loss of work _____

Description of work when rash began _____

_____

_____

_____

_____

Materials contacted at work (new?) _____

_____

_____

_____

Effect of weekends?   Improved _____ Unimproved _____ Worse _____

Effect of vacations?   Improved _____ Unimproved _____ Worse _____

Are other workers affected? No _____ Yes _____ (How many?) _____

Previous compensation claims? No _____ Yes _____

Second job? No _____ Yes _____ (Type) _____

FIGURE 2-1, cont'd
Page 3 of five-part patch test and occupational history and physical examination form.   *Continued*

PATCH TEST AND OCCUPATIONAL HISTORY AND PHYSICAL EXAMINATION

PHYSICAL EXAMINATION

General appearance _____

_____

Description of skin disease _____

_____

_____

_____

SPECIAL TESTS

☐ Potassium hydroxide (KOH)   ☐ Fungal culture   ☐ Bacterial culture

☐ Biopsy _____   ☐ Other tests: _____

FIGURE 2-1, cont'd
Page 4 of five-part patch test and occupational history and physical examination form.   *Continued*

PATCH TEST AND OCCUPATIONAL HISTORY AND PHYSICAL EXAMINATION

Patch Tests ☐ Standard   ☐ Other _____

       ☐ Vehicle and preservative   _____

       ☐ Perfume   _____

                                       _____

Date patch test interpreted _____

Diagnosis _____

_____

_____

RECOMMENDATIONS

PREVENTION

    ☐ Hand eczema sheet

    ☐ Allergen avoidance—exposure list given

    ☐ Protective gloves (Type) _____

TREATMENT

    ☐ Steroids _____

    ☐ Antihistamines _____

    ☐ Other _____

                         _____

Return to work? No _____ Yes _____ Date _____

           Change jobs? No _____ Yes _____

           Restrictions _____

                        _____

FIGURE 2-1, cont'd
Page 5 of five-part patch test and occupational history and physical examination form.

PHYSICAL EXAMINATION

The physical examination should include a total skin examination. Eczematous morphologic appearance and distribution are, of course, the most common findings that raise the index of suspicion for allergic contact dermatitis.

> **"Location is everything."**

In addition to misconceptions about allergic contact dermatitis that are held by patients, there are also misconceptions that physicians have been taught about allergic contact dermatitis. These relate to physical findings as well as history. Some of the frequent ones that can lead to a low level of suspicion and failure to patch test are listed in Table 2-4. Contact dermatitis is *not* always equal in severity bilaterally; it *can* involve the palms and soles. In addition, many of us hold some of the same misconceptions as our patients (see Table 2-3).

The physical examination is a routine one for the dermatologist. It is essential to examine the entire skin surface. Many times the true distribution of an eruption can reveal the antigen source for a patient who for any number of reasons has not given full information on the history. Remember that urticarial and dermal reactions, as well as generalized dermatitis, can represent contact allergy.

MANAGEMENT

Before Patch Testing

Once the history and physical examination are completed and a contact allergy is suspected, patch testing should be performed. Chapter 3 deals with the techniques for testing. It may not be feasible or desirable to patch test at the time of the decision to proceed to testing. The patient must receive treatment, however, until testing is performed.

Treatment consists of removing possible sources of antigens and control of disease. The patient should be instructed to stop using topical medications and personal care products presently being used in the area of involvement. For example, a patient with hand dermatitis need not stop using facial makeup but should discontinue presently used topical medication and hand lotions. Patients with eyelid and facial dermatitis should discontinue using all facial cosmetics and remove nail polish, artificial nails, and nail wraps. Occupationally related dermatitis may necessitate staying away from work (see Chapter 14). Photosensitive patients should avoid sun exposure. Of particular concern is the patient with contact urticaria, since such patients can develop anaphylaxis on exposure to the antigen.

> **Interim treatment before patch testing includes instruction in avoidance of possible antigens and local care.**

Treatment should be as for any case of dermatitis. Acute lesions benefit from cool water soaks. Topical corticosteroids without preservatives (such as **Synalar,**

Aristocort, or **Diprosone ointments**) should be prescribed. Prescribing a topical agent with a preservative in a preservative-allergic patient adds "insult to injury." If corticosteroid allergy is considered possible, either the class of steroid should be changed or the patient should be treated with an alternative immunomodulator like Protopic. Even antihistamine therapy should be tailored to avoid giving diphenhydramine HCl (Benadryl) to a patient who has been sensitized to diphenhydramine HCl in a calamine base (Caladryl) or tripelennamine to an ethylenediamine-sensitive patient. Systemic corticosteroids can, of course, be used in severe cases, but this may delay patch testing.

> **Involving the patient in the workup of allergic contact dermatitis can assist both the clinician and the patient. Patient education is essential to this process.**

Remember, when taking the history and readying for patch testing, that the evaluation and treatment of allergic contact dermatitis can be one of the most exciting and rewarding processes in all of dermatology, especially if the patient is involved actively in the process.

After Patch Testing

The post–patch test visit is the most important part of the process of evaluation and management. An extended block of time should be scheduled so as not to rush through this important part of the disease management process. Once the physician has identified chemicals to which he or she believes the patient is allergic, the physician must determine their relevance to the patient's problem. This means that he or she must identify an exposure source of that allergen in the patient's environment and confirm that the allergen contacted the area of dermatitis *(clinical relevance).*

This textbook is designed to assist in the process just described. Each antigen is listed in a single area of the book with an exposure list. Once the source or sources of antigen inducing the present problem are identified, the patient should be given suggestions for alternatives and methods of avoiding future contact with the antigen. We suggest giving copies of exposure lists to the patient.

> **Give a copy of the exposure list for each allergen of significance to the patient.**

Management of the patient with no relevant positive reactions is more difficult. Either there is an allergic contact dermatitis and an apparently irrelevant positive response is in fact relevant, the causative antigen was not tested, the causative antigen resulted in a false-negative response for various reasons outlined in the next chapter, or the patient does not have an allergic contact dermatitis. A thorough review of exposure lists for positive patch test findings that enlists the patient's aid often reveals a covert source. A careful review of the history to elicit possible untested allergens may be useful but less likely in the patient tested to relevant trays. Reexamination for possible factors leading to a false-negative test result, including undertaking a use test (repeat open application test [ROAT]) of highly suspect products, is recommended.

When all fails, the patient should be managed for a time as having an "other dermatitis," and if control is impossible, the whole process should be reexamined.

CHAPTER 3

Patch Testing

Seventy years ago Sulzberger and Wise (1931) formally introduced patch testing to the American dermatologic community. The authors presented data on more than 100 patients with eczema in whom this technique was used and identified relevant positive reactions in more than 50% of those tested.

> **In this condition (eczema, dermatitis) the contact or patch test should be employed, for it, and it alone, can aid in the quest of the etiologic factor and in the study of the dermatitis.**
> **Sulzberger and Wise, 1931**

The technique was initially devised 35 years earlier by Jadassohn. Great strides have been made in our understanding of the mechanisms of allergic contact dermatitis since the early 1900s, and from time to time various in vitro assays have shown promise as methods of detecting sensitivity to contact allergens. Still, the patch test is the only scientific proof of contact allergy.

> **Properly applied and correctly interpreted patch tests are, at present, the only scientific "proof" of allergic contact dermatitis.**
>
> **Fisher, 1986**

Despite the high prevalence of allergic contact dermatitis among our patients and the fact that diagnostic patch testing is essential to the care and management of these individuals, this simple bioassay is sorely underutilized. A recent survey of members of the American Academy of Dermatology revealed that 27% of respondents did *no* patch testing in their practices. Since 58% of members were nonresponders, the percentage of dermatologists who do not patch test is probably even higher and may approach 50%. The percentages of other groups of clinicians who care for patients with dermatitis, including allergists, occupational medicine physicians, family practitioners, and pediatricians who do not patch test, are certainly even larger.

> **Education in the technique of patch testing is as essential to physicians in training as the learning of most surgical procedures.**
>
> **Fisher, 1986**

Training in the technique is essential to proper use. As in all of medicine, learning is a lifelong continuum. Being trained in the technique of patch testing includes the following:

1. Developing an understanding of the pathophysiology of allergic contact dermatitis
2. Developing a high index of suspicion for the diagnosis of allergic contact dermatitis so as to properly choose patients to be tested
3. Learning the technical application of the test: what you need and where to get it, how and when to apply the test, and how to read the test
4. Developing expertise in determining the relevance of a positive test result and instruction of the patient in avoidance of the allergen

As the clinician uses the patch test, he or she becomes more learned in all aspects of the technique. Almost every application of the test is a learning experience for the physician. Although improper usage can lead to both underdiagnosis and overdiagnosis of contact allergy, each with different and potentially serious consequences, the greatest abuse of patch testing is failure to use the test.

> **The greatest abuse of patch testing is failure to use the test.**
>
> **Colman, 1982**

Learning the basics is best accomplished during residency training. If patch testing techniques are not taught during those years, physicians should avail themselves of continuing medical education training courses available through national organizations, particularly the American Academy of Dermatology (AAD) and the American Contact Dermatitis Society (ACDS). The latter organization meets annually in conjunction with the AAD and additionally sponsors regional meetings that deal with the scientific and practical aspects of diagnosing and caring for individuals with contact dermatitis. Information about the ACDS can be obtained at ACDS, 930 N. Meacham Road, Schaumburg, IL 60173-6016 or at their web site—www.contactderm.org.

If courses and scientific meetings are not available to the physician, the basics can be learned through the use of texts, audiovisual materials, or both, dealing specifically with patch testing.

This textbook is designed to assist the novice in learning basic techniques, regardless of availability of other materials. Further, it is meant to assist in the ongoing learning process that occurs as the physician uses the technique. The more one tests, the more one learns about allergic contact dermatitis and about patch testing.

> **Just do it.**
>
> Cher, 1990

Chapters 1 and 2 deal with understanding the pathophysiology of contact dermatitis and choosing the patient to patch test, respectively. This chapter deals with learning the techniques for application and reading of the patch test; this and the following chapters (Chapters 5 to 11) deal with determining the relevance of positive test results and instruction of the patient in avoidance of allergens.

ALLERGENS AND APPARATUSES

To begin patch testing, the clinician needs antigens. The antigens are available in two forms. In the first, they are supplied to the clinician and dispensed in vehicles to be placed in small aluminum chambers (Finn chambers). This system utilizes antigens in small syringes and dropper bottles and will be referred to as the *Finn Chamber System Test Kit*. It was previously known as the *Allergen Patch Test Kit* (Center Labs). In the second system the antigens are already dispensed in a polymer base (T.R.U.E. Test system).

> **Apparatuses for patch testing include antigens (either T.R.U.E. Test or the Finn Chamber System Test Kit), Finn chambers, Scanpor tape, a skin marker, and record sheets.**

The T.R.U.E. Test system presently consists of 23 or 24 antigens. The other system of antigens, the Finn Chamber System Test Kit marketed for the United States, consists of a standard tray of 20 antigens. Many more antigens of this type are available in Europe and Canada. Regardless of which system the clinician chooses, Finn chambers and Scanpor tape are needed for testing of nonstandard allergens. In addition, a skin marker and record sheets are needed.

The patch test is a biologic assay fraught with individual variability. All aspects of the test that can be standardized should be. Although other systems for applying the antigens, such as A1-test strips, have been used and antigens can be applied with "Band-Aids" and the like, we strongly recommend use of Finn chambers and Scanpor tape.

After removal of the patches two readings must be done, one on removal and a second reading 1 or more days later. The application sites are marked so that readings can be done at the later times. The markings must remain visible for the second reading. A number of systems are available to mark the skin, but no marking system is perfect. The two most frequently used are felt-tipped permanent markers and fluorescent marking pens or paint. The latter is cumbersome because it requires a fluorescent light source for reading. On the other hand, the former can be rubbed off and may stain clothing. A marking system is supplied with the T.R.U.E. Test system.

A record sheet should be used for all readings. Such sheets are available with the standard-tray antigens. For other antigens we recommend a homemade six-column sheet that can be inserted in the patient's chart (Figure 3-1). The columns should include the following (1) number, (2) antigen, (3) first, and (4) second patch test morphology readings, (5) patch-test interpretation, and (6) clinical relevance determination.

In the recent past, professionally prepared allergens have been difficult to obtain in the United States. The Food and Drug Administration has imposed requirements of quality control and proof of efficacy and safety for patch test antigens similar to requirements for marketing of other pharmaceutical agents. This ensures quality antigens for patch testing, but the result of such regulatory oversight has been a paucity of antigens sold in this country because of the high cost of increased premarketing testing and more stringent manufacturing techniques. Presently only the Finn Chamber System Test Kit of 20 allergens and the 23- or 24-allergen T.R.U.E. Test system are available for purchase in the United States (Figure 3-2). Many other antigens are available from European manufacturers but are not legally sold within the United States. However, the use of such antigens by the clinician to patch test patients in the United States is not illegal.

> **Only 20 to 24 patch test antigens are sold within the United States. Patch testing with other antigens, however, is not illegal.**

Most of the antigens discussed in this book are available from a number of sources. In Chapter 5, Table 5-2 we have listed contact information about the major companies that sell these products. Sources for the standard trays for T.R.U.E. Test and the Finn Chamber System Test Kit, Finn chambers, Scanpor tape, and marking systems are also listed. These companies frequently have exhibits at national medical society meetings as well. As an alternative, raw chemicals can be purchased from chemical supply companies and mixed at appropriate concentrations in proper vehicles by a pharmacist or chemist.

Antigen Concentration and Vehicle

The antigens listed in this textbook and sold by the manufacturers listed in Table 5-2 are standardized as to concentration and vehicle. Such standardization has generally been achieved from years of testing large numbers of individuals who were allergic to each antigen, as well as individuals who acted as normal controls. The basis of this standardization is an attempt to balance sensitivity and specificity of the biologic assay—the patch test for the given antigen. Using such standard antigens should result in positive test results in the vast majority of allergic individuals

PATCH TEST RECORD SHEET

Patient Name _____ # _____

Application Date _____

#	Antigen	Morphology Reading		Interpretation	Clinical Relevance
		1st Date	2nd Date		

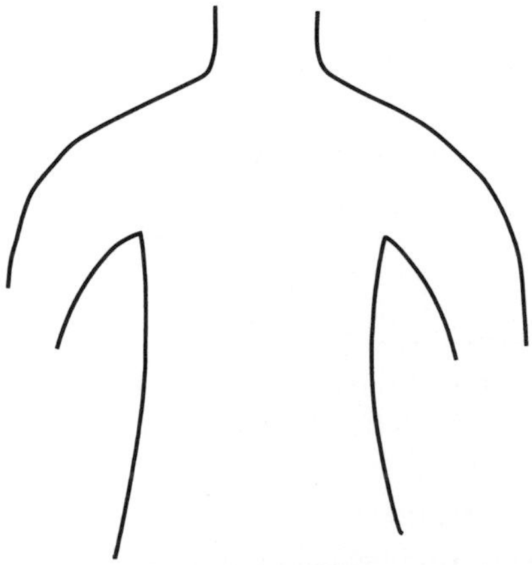

Codes

Morphology	Interpretation		Relevance
+/−	ALL	Allergic	Present
+	?	Unknown	Past
++	IRR	Irritant	Unknown
+++	−	Negative	Not Tested
IRR	NT	Not Tested	
−			
NT			

Application Sites

FIGURE 3-1
Patch test record sheet.

Most topical medic
like anthralin and wart
  If a clothing, shoe,
should be removed and
dose vials) and applied
cations of such produc
tive response in an alle

**A positive respons
controls (5 to 10 in**

In addition, a positi
components to identify

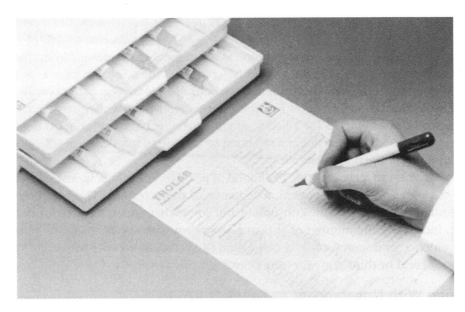

FIGURE 3-2
Standard allergen patch test tray with a recording form. (Courtesy Hermal Pharmaceutical Laboratories.)

and few positive test findings in controls, that is, the fewest false-negative and false-positive results possible for a given allergen. The most common cause for false-positive responses is irritation. Such reactions are due primarily to too high a concentration but may also be affected by the vehicle.

In addition, the concentrations of the standardized antigens should not actively produce sensitization in tested individuals. It is recommended that the clinician use standardized, commercially available antigens whenever possible. For less common antigens the reader is referred to deGroot (1986).

Which antigens to use for testing in a particular patient depend on the history and the distribution of the eruption. This is called directed or aimed antigen selection. Even the best clinician, however, can be fooled, and the novice is even more likely to choose incorrectly. For this reason, we do not recommend strict **directed** antigen selection. Our approach is more "shotgun" or tray-selected testing. This usually results in testing larger numbers of antigens. It has been suggested that such testing can increase the incidence of "angry back" or "excited skin syndrome" and false-positive results. We believe that such a risk is greatly outweighed by the increase in the probability of testing to the relevant antigens that could otherwise be missed.

All patients should be tested to a **standard series,** either the Finn Chamber System Test Kit or the T.R.U.E. Test. The antigens in those kits are the most frequent agents causing allergic contact dermatitis in the general population in the country where marketed. Frequently, positive reactions are found that do not relate to the present dermatitis (no **present relevance**) but relate to previous exposures **(past relevance).** Such information given to the patient with proper education in avoidance may be important preventive medicine.

All patients should be tested to a standard series.

DETERMINING CLINICAL RELEVANCE

Most important, once a positive allergic reaction is documented for an allergen, clinical relevance must be determined (Table 3-5). Such a determination is based on the history and an understanding of the sources of the antigen in the patient's environment. The clinician should refer to the specific antigen sections in this textbook that focus on the exposure lists for the positive antigens. These lists contain three parts: synonyms and other names, common uses of the antigens, and tips on prevention of exposure. We recommend giving a copy of the list to the patient.

> **The exposure lists in this textbook should be used for both determining the clinical relevance of a positive reaction and for assisting the patient in allergen avoidance.**

Relevance of reactions may be **present,** that is, the cause or at least an aggravating factor in the present dermatitis, or **past,** that is, the cause of a previous dermatitis. Even after extensive investigations there may be no evidence of relevance **(unknown).** In such cases the patient should still be given the exposure lists and should be instructed to avoid contact with the antigen. Occasionally the patient recognizes a source of exposure and positive relevance only after going over the list again at home.

INSTRUCTION OF PATIENTS IN AVOIDANCE OF ALLERGENS

In addition to explaining the exposure list to the patient, the physician should make suggestions for substitutions of products that do not contain the allergen. Such tips as to prevention are given in each exposure list.

The exposure list has the following purposes:
1. To assist the physician in determining relevance
2. To assist the physician in instructing the patient in future antigen avoidance

For further discussion of antigen avoidance in the workplace the reader is referred to Chapter 14.

> **Exposure lists for each positive test antigen should be given to the patient and discussed in the office of the physician. It must be stressed that such lists are not absolutely complete but are general guidelines.**

Table 3-5	Clinical Relevance*
	Present
	Past
	Unknown

*See Figure 3-1.

Negative Patch Test Results

Negative patch test results can mean either that no allergy exists as a cause of the patient's dermatitis or that there was a failure of the patch test—a false-negative response.

False-negative responses can be due to a number of situations, the most prominent of which are the following:

1. *Failure to test for a response to the proper antigen.* Careful retaking of the history and testing with products from the environment may reveal the true culprit. Failure to recognize and test for photoallergy also results in negative results, even with proper antigen choice.
2. *Testing with too low a concentration of proper antigen.* Higher concentrations, alternative vehicles, or even slightly different chemical structures for given antigens can be used when the history strongly suggests that an antigen is causal. We refer the readers to more encyclopedic reference texts for assistance.
3. *Improper testing technique.* If all the suggested techniques have been followed (e.g., 48 hours' contact of the patch; a second, delayed reading; and proper patient preparation), this situation does not usually occur.

If after review, the clinician believes that the patch test result is truly negative, the patient should be told that no contact allergy can presently be identified. It should be stressed, however, that there are limitations to testing and that retesting at a future date might be indicated.

Repeat Open Application Test

The repeat open application test (ROAT) is used primarily in the clinical setting of a negative patch test result associated with a strong suspicion of allergic contact dermatitis. The suspected antigen is usually a component of a personal care product or a topical medicament. When the patient and/or physician believes that the product is responsible for the dermatitis and when closed patch test results to the product are negative, a ROAT may be indicated. In such cases the result of testing with components of the product is also usually negative. In some cases, however, test results to the product are negative, despite a positive response to a component tested alone. For example, testing with the standard-tray antigens reveals a positive reaction to a preservative, and the preservative is present in the moisturizer used by the patient; however, the result of a patch test to the moisturizer is negative. In the ROAT the patient is instructed to apply the product to a localized body site (usually one antecubital fossa), once or twice a day for 1 week. This usually produces a localized dermatitis that confirms the suspected allergy. Such testing may cause a flare-up of a more generalized dermatitis and therefore should be approached with care.

Side Effects of Patch Testing

Patch testing to antigens at standard concentration and in standard vehicles is an extremely safe procedure. However, adverse reactions can occur. One of the most frequent is flare-up of the contact dermatitis with a positive test reaction to the relevant antigen. This may actually provide a clue to the clinician that the patch test is relevant. Severe reactions (allergic or irritant) can lead in rare cases to scarring, hypopigmentation, or hyperpigmentation. Occasionally, persistent reactions or bacterial or viral infections can occur.

CHAPTER 5

Standard Allergens

AMMONIATED MERCURIC CHLORIDE (CHAPTER 6)
BLACK RUBBER MIX (*N*-ISOPROPYL-*N*ᴵ-PHENYL-
  p-PHENYLENEDIAMINE)
CAINE MIX (BENZOCAINE)
CARBA MIX
COBALT DICHLORIDE
COLOPHONY
EPOXY RESIN
ETHYLENEDIAMINE DIHYDROCHLORIDE
FORMALDEHYDE
FRAGRANCE MIXTURE
IMIDAZOLIDINYL UREA
LANOLIN ALCOHOL
MERCAPTO MIX
MERCAPTOBENZOTHIAZOLE
METHYLCHLOROISOTHIAZOLINONE/
  METHYLISOTHIAZOLINONE
MYROXYLON PEREIRAE (BALSAM OF PERU)
NEOMYCIN SULFATE
NICKEL
p-PHENYLENEDIAMINE
p-tert-BUTYLPHENOL FORMALDEHYDE RESIN
PARABEN MIX
POTASSIUM DICHROMATE
PRIMIN
QUATERNIUM-15
QUINOLINE MIX
SESQUITERPENE LACTONE MIX
THIMEROSAL
THIURAM MIX
URUSHIOL (CHAPTER 10)

The standard-tray or screening series allergens should be viewed as the starting point for patch testing all patients suspected of having allergic contact dermatitis. These antigens are the most common causes of allergic contact dermatitis in the general population and serve initially as an excellent screen for contact allergy. Since the patient's history often does not give clues to the origin or cause of the contact dermatitis or can be misleading, it is recommended that every patient be tested with the entire standard tray. Frequently, unexpected positive patch test reactions occur and lead to the correct diagnosis and identification of the putative allergen. For example, many patients with a cosmetic allergy are misdiagnosed unless the entire standard tray is applied, which may reveal an allergy to a preservative or fragrance within the offending cosmetic. The history of cosmetic use is often misleading or not helpful until a specific allergen is identified; then the patient looks for exposure to that allergen in his or her cosmetics. Thus we recommend that most patients have the entire standard series applied to avoid otherwise unfound allergens. In addition, frequent use of the standard tray gives the clinician experience with the performance of the individual allergens. For example, formaldehyde, which is used at a near-irritant concentration, can cause questionable macular erythematous reactions. These reactions can generally be ignored.

> **The standard tray is the starting point. Test every patient with the entire standard tray, and test additional allergens when appropriate.**

The standard tray is sometimes insufficient for discovering the allergen responsible for allergic contact dermatitis (Box 5-1). In selected patients, additional allergens are tested in a more directed manner. For example, the patient's occupation may warrant testing with more allergens. A hairdresser should be tested with

---

BOX 5-1

Supplemental Allergens for the Standard Tray

You may want to patch test everyone with extra allergens in addition to the standard tray. For example:

Preservatives
2-Bromo-2 nitropropane-1, 3 diol
Imidazolidinyl urea
Diazolidinyl urea
DMDM hydantoin

Rubber Compound
Thiourea

Textiles
Disperse Blue 106
Ethyleneurea/melamine formaldehyde
 resin

Medicaments
Bacitricin
Tixocortol-21-pivalate
Budesonide

Cosmetics
Tosylamide/formaldehyde resin
Ethyl acrylate
Glyceryl thioglycolate

Miscellaneous
Thimerosal
Sodium gold thiosulfate

glyceryl thioglycolate, the allergen in acid permanent-wave solutions, in addition to the standard tray. Other occupations require specific allergens depending on the chemicals used in their industry. The distribution of dermatitis might also warrant further testing. A sun-exposed distributed dermatitis suggests a photoallergic contact dermatitis requiring photo–patch testing with photoallergens. But the standard tray should not be overlooked, since the authors have seen patients with typical photo-distributed dermatitis caused by allergic contact dermatitis that is due to an airborne standard allergen. There are different standard series varying on regional preferences. (Tables 5-1 and 5-2). The T.R.U.E. Test and the European and Japanese standard series are presented in this chapter for comparison.

Table 5-1	Standard Allergen Series		
T.R.U.E. Test	European	Japanese	
Medicaments			
Neomycin sulfate	Neomycin sulfate	Neomycin (Fradiomycin)	
Caine mix	Benzocaine	Caine mix	
Quinoline mix*	Clioquinol	Ammoniated mercuric chloride	
Preservatives			
Formaldehyde	Formaldehyde	Formaldehyde	
Quaternium-15	Quaternium-15	Methylchloroisothiazolinone/ methylchloroisothiazolinone	
Methylchloroisothiazolinone/ methylisothiazolinone	Methylchloroisothiazolinone/ methylisothiazolinone	Thimerosal	
Paraben mix	Paraben mix	Paraben mix	
Thimerosal			
Rubber Compounds			
Thiuram mix	Thiuram mix	Thiuram mix	
Mercaptobenzothiazole	Mercaptobenzothiazole	Mercapto mix	
Mercapto mix	Mercapto mix	Dithiocarbamate mix	
Carba mix	N-Isopropyl-N^{l}-phenyl-p- phenylenediamine	Black rubber mix	
Black rubber mix			
Vehicles			
Wool alcohol	Wool alcohol	Lanolin alcohol	
Metals			
Nickel sulfate	Nickel sulfate	Nickel sulfate	
Potassium dichromate	Potassium dichromate	Potassium dichromate	
Cobalt chloride	Cobalt chloride	Cobalt chloride	

*Quinoline mix has been deleted from the T.R.U.E. Test sold in the United States. It remains on the European T.R.U.E. Test.

Continued

Table 5-1

Standard Allergen Series—cont'd

T.R.U.E. Test	European	Japanese
Fragrances		
Balsam of Peru	Balsam of Peru	Balsam of Peru
Fragrance mix	Fragrance mix	Fragrance mix
Resins		
Epoxy	Epoxy	Epoxy
p-tert–Butylphenol formaldehyde	*p-tert*–Butylphenol formaldehyde	*p-tert*–Butylphenol formaldehyde
Miscellaneous		
Colophony	Colophony	Colophony
p-Phenylenediamine	4-Phenylenediamine base	*p*-Phenylenediamine
Ethylenediamine dihydrochloride	Primin	Ethylenediamine dihydrochloride
	Sesquiterpene lactone mix	Primin
		Urushiol
		Petrolatum

Table 5-2

Sources of Allergen

Allerderm Laboratories, Inc.
P.O. Box 2070
Petaluma, CA 94953-2070
Tel: 1-800-365-6868
Fax: 707-664-0666
Web site: www.allerderm.com

Chemotechnique Diagnostics AB
P.O. Box 80, Edvard Ols vag 2
S-230 42 Tygelsjö,
Sweden
Tel: 46-40 46 60 77
Fax: 46 40 46 67 00
E-mail: info@chemotechnique.se

Dormer Laboratories, Inc.
91 Kelfield Street, #5
Rexdale, Ontario M9W 5A3
Tel: 416-242-6167
Fax: 877-430-7637
E-mail: info@dormer.com
Web site: www.dormer.com

Hermal Kurt Herrmann
Scholtzstrasse 3
D-2057 Reinbek
Hamburg, Germany
Tel: 0049/40-72704 0
Fax: 0049/40-722 92 96

Pharmascience, Inc.
8400 ch. Darnley Rd.
CND-Montréal, Québec H4T 1M4
Tel: 0450 458 0158
Fax: 0450 458 1477

BIBLIOGRAPHY

Bruynzeel DP, Andersen KE, Camarasa JG et al: The European standard series, *Contact Dermatitis* 33:145-148, 1995.

Guin JD, editor: *Practical contact dermatitis: a handbook for the practitioner,* New York, 1995, McGraw-Hill.

Isaksson M, Brandao FM, Bruze M et al: Recommendation to include budesonide and tixocortol pivalate in the European standard series, *Contact Dermatitis* 43:41-63, 2000.

James WE, Rosenthal LE, Brancaccio RR, Marks JG: American Academy of Dermatology Patch Testing Survey: use and effectiveness of this procedure, *J Am Acad Dermatol* 26:991-994, 1992.

Lewis FM, Cork MJ, McDonagh AJG, Gawkrodger DJ: An audit of the value of patch testing: the patient's perspective, *Contact Dermatitis* 30:214-216, 1994.

Marks JG, Belsito DV, DeLeo VA et al: North American Contact Dermatitis Group standard tray patch test results: 1992 to 1994, *Am J Contact Dermat* 6:160-165, 1995.

Marks JG, Belsito DV, DeLeo VA et al: North American Contact Dermatitis Group patch test results for the detection of delayed-type hypersensitivity to topical allergens, *J Am Acad Dermatol* 38:911-918, 1998.

Marks JG, Belsito DV, DeLeo VA et al: North American Contact Dermatitis Group standard tray patch test results: 1996 to 1998, *Arch Dermatol* 136:272-273, 2000.

Rietschel RL, Fowler JF: *Fisher's contact dermatitis,* ed 5, Baltimore, 2001, Williams & Wilkins.

Rycroft RJ, Mennè T, Frosch PJ, editors: *Textbook of contact dermatitis,* Berlin, 1995, Springer-Verlag.

Sherertz EF, Swartz SM: Is the screening patch test tray still worth using? *J Am Acad Dermatol* 29:1057-1058, 1993.

BLACK RUBBER MIX (N-ISOPROPYL-Nⁱ-PHENYL-*p*-PHENYLENEDIAMINE)

Definition

Black rubber mix (in T.R.U.E. Test) is tested at a 0.075 mg/cm^2 concentration in polyvidone. It is composed of the following:

N-phenyl-Nⁱ-cyclohexyl-*p*-phenylenediamine (CPPD) 0.0255 mg

N-isopropyl-Nⁱ-phenyl-*p*-phenylenediamine (IPPD) 0.0102 mg

N,Nⁱ-diphenyl-*p*-phenylenediamine (DPPD) 0.0255 mg

In the European standard tray, the black rubber mix mix was replaced with IPPD at 0.1% in petrolatum. However, only testing with IPPD may miss approximately 10% of patients sensitized to these industrial rubber chemicals.

The preceding amines are used as antioxidants and antiozonants in the production of rubber and are the most effective and commonly used of available agents. The compounds prevent drying and cracking of the final rubber products. Since they discolor and stain, they are used primarily in black rubber, where this effect is not noticeable: hence the term *black rubber mix.* In the study from 1996 to 1998 of the North American Dermatitis Group (Marks and others, 2000) 1.5% of patients reacted to IPPD.

Clinical Aspects

The three *p*-phenylenediamine compounds are widely used in the manufacture of rubber, primarily for industrial purposes. Since these agents discolor the final product, most finished products containing these agents are dark, either gray or black. These include tires, tubes, pipes, gaskets, flanges, mail sorters, heavy black rubber gloves and boots, shoes (especially soles), cushions, earphones, and walking-stick

EXPOSURE LIST	CAINE MIX (Benzocaine)

Synonyms and Other Names

Benzocaine
  Aethoform
  Americaine
  p-Aminobenzoic acid (PABA) ethyl ester
  Anesthane
  Anesthesin
  Early aminobenzoate
  Orthesin
  Parathesin

Dibucaine
  Cincaine
  Cinchocaine
  Dibucaine hydrochloride
  Nupercaine
  Percaine
  Sovcaine
Tetracaine
  Cetacaine
  Pontocaine

Uses

Caines are used primarily as a topical anesthetic to reduce itching and pain. They are found in the following products:

1. Burn and sunburn remedies
2. Hemorrhoidal creams, suppositories, and enemas
3. Poison ivy products
4. Oral and gingival products for teething, toothaches, canker sores, and denture irritation and in oral antibacterial agents
5. Sore throat sprays and lozenges
6. Cough tablets, drops, and lozenges
7. Astringents and analgesics
8. Podiatric products for athlete's foot, corns, calluses, and warts
9. Appetite suppressants

Prevention

Patients sensitive to benzocaine should avoid all products claiming topical relief of pain or itching unless the product is clearly labeled and benzocaine and tetracaine are not included. Such agents can be used if they contain *only* dibucaine or lidocaine. Persons sensitive to benzocaine may have a serious reaction to related anesthetic agents derived from benzoic acid when given by injection from dentists, physicians, or other health care workers; such individuals should always be advised of the patient's allergy to benzocaine. Patients should be able to tolerate other chemically unrelated agents without difficulty, including lidocaine and mepivacaine.

Benzocaine- and tetracaine-sensitive individuals may also have to avoid PABA and PABA esters containing sunscreens, permanent hair dye (*p*-phenylenediamine), certain diuretics or fluid pills (hydrochlorothiazide), oral antidiabetic medications (sulfonylureas), certain antibiotics including sulfa drugs (and PAS), azo and aniline dyes, and an important cardiac medication, procainamide (Pronestyl). Allergic persons should always show this list to appropriate health care workers.

Patients who are allergic to caine mix must undergo further testing to determine the component of the mix to which they are allergic. If they are allergic to benzocaine and tetracaine, the preceding recommendations apply. If they are allergic to dibucaine, they must avoid that agent in topical and injectable form and, in addition, should avoid lidocaine, other related amide anesthetics like mepivacaine, and quinoline antiinfectives like iodochlorhydroxyquin.

May be duplicated for use in clinical practice. From Marks JG Jr, Elsner P, DeLeo VA: *Contact and occupational dermatology,* ed 3, St Louis, 2002, Mosby.

Table 5-4	Agents That May Cross-React With Benzocaine
Chemical	**Use**
Procainamide (Pronestyl)	Antiarrhythmic
Hydrochlorothiazide (HydroDiuril)	Diuretic
p-Aminobenzoic acid (PABA) and PABA esters	Sunscreens
Azo and aniline dyes	Dyes
p-Phenylenediamine	Hair and fur dyes
Sulfonamides	Antibiotics
Sulfonylureas (chlorpropamide)	Antidiabetic agents
p-Aminosalicylic acid	Antimicrobial

sensitive to dibucaine, benzocaine, or tetracaine and as such may react to the benzoic acid esters, and to the anilide and amide group, to which the quinolines belong. Therefore it is necessary to follow up a positive caine mix test result with further testing to determine which of the component(s) is (are) the allergen(s). In addition, patients who are sensitive to dibucaine may react to the quinoline anti-infective agents, including iodochlorhydroxyquin (Vioform).

In addition to cross-reactivity within the benzoic acid derivative groups, individuals who are sensitized to benzocaine may also develop a reaction to procainamide, sulfonamides, PABA, sunscreens, p-aminosalicylic acid (PAS), p-phenylenediamine hydrochloride in hair and fur dyes, hydrochlorothiazide diuretics, sulfonylurea oral hypoglycemics, and azo and aniline dyes (Table 5-4).

BIBLIOGRAPHY

Cronin E: *Contact dermatitis,* London, 1980, Churchill Livingstone.

Fisher AA: Allergic reactions to topical anesthetics, *Cutis* 25:584-590, 1980.

Lodi A, Ambonati A, Coassini Z et al: Contact allergy to "caines" caused by antihemorrhoidal ointments, *Contact Dermatitis* 41:221-222, 1999.

Marks JG, Belsito DV, DeLeo VA et al: North American Contact Dermatitis Group standard tray patch test results: 1996 to 1998, *Arch Dermatol* 136:272-273, 2000.

Mathewson HS: *Structural forms of anesthetic compounds,* Kansas City, MO, 1961, Charles C Thomas.

Ryan ME, Davis BM, Marks JG: Contact urticaria and allergic contact dermatitis to benzocaine gel, *J Am Acad Dermatol* 2:221-223, 1980.

Sidhu SK, Shaw S, Wilkinson JD: A 10-year retrospective study on benzocaine allergy in the United Kingdom, *Am J Contact Dermat,* 10:57-61, 1999.

Storrs F, Rosenthal LE, Adams RM et al: Prevalence and relevance of allergic reactions in patients tested in North America: 1984 to 1985, *J Am Acad Dermatol* 20:1038-1044, 1989.

CARBA MIX

Definition

Carba mix is a combination of two dithiocarbamates and a noncarbamate, diphenylguanidine. Each of the following are present at 1% in petrolatum (total 3%) or in the T.R.U.E. Test in equal parts for a total amount of 0.25 mg/cm^2 in hydroxypropyl cellulose:

EXPOSURE LIST	COBALT DICHLORIDE

Synonyms and Other Names
Cobalt
Cobalt blue
Cobaltous (adjective)

Uses
Cobalt is found in many metallic items as well as a number of nonmetallic sources, including the following:
1. Jewelry
2. Snaps, zippers, buttons, and buckles
3. Tools, utensils, and instruments
4. Machinery parts
5. Vitamin B_{12}
6. Hair dyes and cosmetics
7. Pigments in pottery, glass, and crayons
8. Joint replacements and dental appliances
9. Shell splinters
10. Cement, paint, and resins
11. Printing inks
12. Tattoos
13. Welding rods
14. Electroplating
15. Animal feed
16. Tires

Prevention
Patients allergic to cobalt should minimize contact with almost any metallic object, particularly jewelry. Substitutes include stainless steel and plastic earrings, necklaces, and so forth.

Allergic patients should also check their cosmetics and hair dyes for the presence of cobalt by reading the labels. Many substitutes are available.

May be duplicated for use in clinical practice. From Marks JG Jr, Elsner P, DeLeo VA: *Contact and occupational dermatology,* ed 3, St Louis, 2002, Mosby.

Cobalt is used primarily in combination with other metals in hard metal alloys. The other metals used in these alloys include nickel, chromium, molybdenum, and tungsten. This usage of cobalt is due to its addition of strength or hardness to alloys, which allows them to resist heat and moisture. Such alloys include Stellite, Vitallium, alnico, duralium, mobilium, Permalloy, and ticonium. These alloys are widely used in such diverse products as human artificial joints and dental implants and jet engines and rockets.

Various salts of cobalt are colored and are used as pigments in colored glass and pottery as well as in makeup and hair dyes.

Cobalt is present in European cement. It is used as a paint drier, in the production of resins, and in nickel-plated objects.

In addition to alloys in which cobalt is synthetically combined with nickel and chromium, cobalt is found in association with both of these metals in nature. This is thought to be the mechanism of frequently combined sensitivity to cobalt and nickel or chromates. This is a cosensitivity, not a cross-sensitivity. Approximately

80% of individuals who are sensitive to cobalt are also found to be sensitive to either chromate or nickel, or both. In men the usual cosensitizer is chromate. This is probably due to the combined presence of chromate and cobalt in cement and other construction-related exposure sources. Women are more frequently cosensitive to cobalt and nickel, as in a jewelry allergy.

Sensitization to cobalt is usually associated with cosensitization to nickel or chromate, or both.

Sensitization to nickel or chromate (or both) in conjunction with active dermatitis appears to predispose to sensitization to cobalt.

Nonoccupational exposure to cobalt includes jewelry; metal components of clothes, such as buttons, snaps, clasps, and buckles; hair dye and antiperspirants; joint replacements and dental appliances; hobby materials including pottery, glass, shell working, and crayons; and vitamin B_{12} injection or ingestion.

Industrial exposure can occur in hard metal industries, tool and die making, hand etching and grinding, polyester resin manufacture, the paint industry, the cement industry, the carbide industry, pottery workers, dentistry, and the manufacture of alloys.

Patch testing with cobalt chloride may yield an unusual false-positive response consisting of tiny purpuric papules.

BIBLIOGRAPHY

Cronin E: *Contact dermatitis,* London, 1980, Churchill Livingstone.

Fischer A, Rystedt I: Cobalt allergy in hand metal workers, *Contact Dermatitis* 9:115, 1983.

Flint GN: A metallurgical approach to metal contact dermatitis, *Contact Dermatitis* 39:213-221, 1998.

Kanerva L, Jolanki R, Estlander T et al: Incidence rates of occupational allergic contact dermatitis caused by metals, *Am J Contact Dermat* 11:155-160, 2000.

Marks JG, Belsito DV, DeLeo VA et al: North American Contact Dermatitis Group standard tray patch test results: 1996 to 1998, *Arch Dermatol* 136:272-273, 2000.

Mueller R, Breucker G: Cobalt as work-dependent eczematogen and as co-allergen with chromium and nickel, *Dermatol Wochenschr* 154:276, 1968.

COLOPHONY (Rosin)

Definition

Colophony (rosin) is a yellow, complex, natural residue left after distilling off the volatile oil from oleoresin obtained from the coniferous tree *Pinus palustris* and from other pine tree species in the family *Pinaceae.* Colophony is patch tested as a 20% concentration in petrolatum, not less than 70% of which is abietic acid, or as 0.85 mg/cm² in hydroxypropyl cellulose in the T.R.U.E. Test. The North American Contact Dermatitis Group found that 2.0% of their patients had positive patch test reactions to this material (Marks and others, 2000).

Colophonium is the name used on cosmetics.

MERCAPTOBENZOTHIAZOLE

Definition

Mercaptobenzothiazole (MBT) is a thiazole rubber accelerator—an agent used to speed up the vulcanization process of cross-linking polymer chains. It is one of the five rubber components or mixtures used in the standard tray. MBT is patch tested at a 1% concentration in petrolatum or 0.075 mg/cm^2 in polyvidone in the T.R.U.E. Test. It resulted in positive patch test responses in 1.8% of patients tested by the North American Contact Dermatitis group (Marks and others, 2000).

> **Mercaptobenzothiazole is a rubber accelerator.**

Clinical Aspects

MBT and other thiazoles are the most common accelerators used in the production of rubber. In addition, MBT has been used in cutting oils, antifreeze, industrial greases, anticorrosive agents, cements and adhesives, detergents, and fungicides. It is used in veterinary products like flea and tick sprays and powders and in photographic film emulsions.

The rate of sensitivity to MBT in patch test clinic patients varies among countries and ranges from 1% to 8%. The thiazoles and the thiurams are routinely found to be the two most common rubber components producing positive patch test responses in such groups.

The most common sources of sensitizing exposure to MBT and other rubber components are gloves and shoes. Shoe contact dermatitis is primarily due to a rubber component allergy, usually MBT and, less frequently, thiurams. A positive MBT allergy in association with a foot dermatitis may be due to rubber shoes such as sneakers or to leather shoes with rubber insoles, box toes, linings, or adhesives used to hold various components together. Usually the dermatitis is limited to the area of contact. This may be primarily the soles of the feet bilaterally, but patients with such an allergy may also have unilateral involvement. In addition, with wear, allergens frequently leach from the offending shoe component and spread to other areas of the shoe. MBT is the most commonly identified allergen in allergic contact dermatitis due to shoes in the United States and accounts for 15% to 45% of positive patch test responses in patients tested in various series for shoe dermatitis.

> **Mercaptobenzothiazole is the most common cause of allergic contact dermatitis from shoes.**

MBT is second to the thiurams as the etiologic agent in allergic contact dermatitis due to gloves. Other rubber sources of exposure to MBT include rubberized fabrics in clothing like brassieres and girdles. While the distribution of the dermatitis commonly involves all areas contacted by the offending rubber, it should be remembered that patchy or unilateral dermatitis of the feet or hands due to shoes or gloves does occur.

Occupational contact dermatitis due to a rubber component allergy is not uncommon and accounts for approximately a quarter of rubber-sensitive patients in some large groups.

EXPOSURE LIST ▷ MERCAPTOBENZOTHIAZOLE

Synonyms and Other Names

2-Benzathiazalethiol	Mertax
Captax	Nocceler M
Dermacid	Rotax
MBT	Thiotax

Uses

MBT is primarily used as a rubber accelerator and therefore may be present in any natural or synthetic rubber products such as the following:

1. Rubber shoes (sneakers and tennis shoes)
2. Leather shoes (insoles and adhesive linings)
3. Gloves (household, work, or hospital)
4. Sponge makeup applicators and rubber eyelash curlers
5. Rubber in undergarments and clothing, diapers
6. Rubber pillows and sheets
7. Condoms and diaphragms
8. Medical devices
9. Swimwear
10. Tires and tubes
11. Toys
12. Renal dialysis equipment

Other, nonrubber sources of exposure include the following:

1. Cutting oils
2. Antifreeze
3. Greases
4. Anticorrosive agents
5. Cements and adhesives
6. Detergents
7. Fungicides
8. Veterinary products such as tick and flea powders and sprays
9. Photographic film emulsion

Prevention

If patients are mercaptobenzothiazole sensitive and have foot dermatitis, it is probably due to their shoes (see Box 5-2). They may wear all-leather shoes with no inner or outer sole, like moccasins. Molded plastic shoes or wooden clogs can be worn. Patients should contact their local shoe stores and ask for U.S.-made, rubber-free shoes. If they cannot find such shoes, the insoles from piano felt, cork, or plastic should be inserted. Sweating should be minimal, and old socks that may contain allergens should be discarded.

Patients who are MBT sensitive and have hand dermatitis should avoid rubber (latex) gloves and, if possible, wear vinyl gloves only (see Box 5-3). If rubber gloves must be worn, manufacturers should be contacted to acquire MBT-free gloves. One important resource that can be contacted if the patient has persistent difficulties is the Allerderm Laboratories, Inc., P.O. Box 2070, Petaluma, California 94953. Call 1-800-365-6868 or visit them at www.allerderm.com.

Allergic patients should avoid contact with other rubber products as listed earlier and check the chemicals used in their work if they are in the agricultural or photographic industries.

May be duplicated for use in clinical practice. From Marks JG Jr, Elsner P, DeLeo VA: *Contact and occupational dermatology,* ed 3, St Louis, 2002, Mosby.

BIBLIOGRAPHY

Cronin E: *Contact dermatitis,* London, 1980, Churchill Livingstone.

Feinman SE: Sensitivity to rubber chemicals, *J Toxicol–Cut Ocular Toxicol* 6(2):117-153, 1987.

Guin JD: The MBT controversy, *Am J Contact Dermat* 1:195-197, 1990.

Marks JG, Belsito DV, DeLeo VA et al: North American Contact Dermatitis Group standard tray patch test results: 1996 to 1998, *Arch Dermatol* 136:272-273, 2000.

Storrs F, Rosenthal LE, Adams RM et al: Prevalence and relevance of allergic reactions in patients tested in North America, *J Am Acad Dermatol* 20:1038-1044, 1989.

METHYLCHLOROISOTHIAZOLINONE/METHYLISOTHIAZOLINONE

Definition

Methylchloroisothiazolinone/methylisothiazolinone (MCI/MI) is a preservative mixture of two isothiazolinones used in cosmetics and industry. It is patch tested as 100 ppm active ingredient in water or 0.0040 mg/cm^2 in polyvidone in the T.R.U.E. Test. The North American Contact Dermatitis Group found 2.9% of its patients to be allergic to this compound (Marks and others, 2000).

> **Methylchloroisothiazolinone/methylisothiazolinone (Kathon) is an important biocide that is used in cosmetics and in industry.**

Clinical Aspects

MCI/MI is a preservative mixture of 1.15% MCI and 0.35% MI in water plus 23% magnesium chloride and nitrate as stabilizers. It is effective at quite low concentrations in controlling the growth of bacteria and fungi. Recommended levels of preservation by the manufacturer are 3 to 15 ppm as active ingredients (0.02% to 0.1% by weight). Allergic contact dermatitis due to MCI/MI was first recognized in Europe, where it was introduced in the mid-1970s. Subsequently, since the early 1980s, it has been used as a cosmetic preservative in the United States. It has a wide range of compatibility with cosmetic ingredients and a broad spectrum of activity against bacterial and fungal organisms. The Cosmetic Ingredient Review expert panel approved maximum concentrations of 7.5 ppm MCI/MI in leave-on products such as moisturizing creams and 15 ppm in rinse-off products such as shampoos. Japan and European Economic Community countries have adopted a maximum concentration in cosmetics of 15 ppm with use limited to rinse-off products in Japan. In 1977, no MCI/MI was used in U.S. cosmetic formulations. By 1993, however, MCI/MI was the tenth most frequently used preservative in cosmetic formulations (1042 products) disclosed to the U.S. Food and Drug Administration.

A rapid increase in allergic contact dermatitis caused by MCI/MI was reported in some European countries. This was in contrast to the experience in North America. Patch test clinics in Europe had an average rate of 3% positive test responses varying from 0.4% in England to 11.0% in Italy. The reasons for the variation in prevalence rates among patch test clinics are complex. One important reason is that varying amounts of preservative were used in different products, with excessive amounts of MCI/MI used in some countries. Interestingly, Frosch and others (1995) showed that most individuals who are sensitive to MCI/MI can use shampoo preserved with MCI/MI without developing allergic contact dermatitis.

Standard Allergens ■ **107**

EXPOSURE LIST	METHYLCHLOROISOTHIAZOLINONE/METHYLISOTHIAZOLINONE

Synonyms and Other Names

Acticide	Kathon DP
Algucid CH50	Kathon UT
Amerstat 250	Kathon LX
Cl + Me—isothizolinone	Metat GT
Euxyl K 100	Metatin GT
Grotan TK-2	Paretol
Kathon WT	Parmetol
Kathon 886 MW	5-Chloro-2-methyl-4-isothiazolin-3-one and
Kathon CG	2-methyl-4-isothiazolin-3-one

Uses

Methylchloroisothiazolinone/methylisothiazolinone (MCI/MI) is a preservative found in cosmetics and medications and used for industrial applications. The following are among the products in which MCI/MI can be found:

1. Cosmetics (shampoos may be tolerated, since they are rinsed off)
2. Household cleaning products
3. Metalworking fluids
4. Latex emulsions and paints
5. Cooling tower water
6. Slime control in paper mills
7. Jet fuels
8. Milk sampling
9. Radiography
10. Printing inks
11. Moist toilet paper
12. Medicated creams, ointments, and the like
13. Adhesives and glue
14. Flax spinning

Prevention

Avoidance of cosmetics containing this allergen is accomplished by reading cosmetic labels. If the ingredients are not listed, a small amount of the cosmetic product should be applied to a small area of skin on the forearm twice daily for 1 week to test for allergic contact dermatitis. In the industrial setting the materials safety data sheets should be examined for sources of exposure. Skin protective measures or a job change may be required.

May be duplicated for use in clinical practice. From Marks JG Jr, Elsner P, DeLeo VA: *Contact and occupational dermatology,* ed 3, St Louis, 2002, Mosby.

Potential explanations for this are that the use concentration of MCI/MI is below the elicitation threshold or the contact time is too short.

Isothiazolinones (Kathon preparations) have also caused allergic contact dermatitis and chemical burns in the workplace. Nethercott and others (1990) found that 11 (41%) of 27 metalworkers with eczematous dermatitis in an engine parts manufacturing plant developed allergic contact dermatitis due to Kathon 886 MW in metalworking fluids. Madden and others (1994) reported machinists in a jet turbine manufacturing plant who developed allergic contact dermatitis to MCI/MI in metalworking fluids. Bruze and others (1990) documented chemical burns and allergic contact dermatitis from accidental exposure to Kathon WT,

---

EXPOSURE LIST	NEOMYCIN SULFATE

Synonyms and Other Names

Fradiomycin (Japan)
Framycetin
Myacine
Mycifradin
Neodecyllin
Neolate
Neomas

Neomin
Neomycin undecylenate
Nivemycin
Pimavecort
Soframycin
Vonamycin Powder V

Uses

Neomycin is the most commonly used antibiotic in skin creams and ointments and in drops used in the eyes and ears. Frequently used in combination with other antibacterials, antifungals, and corticosteroids, neomycin is available in prescription and nonprescription forms and is infrequently used by dentists and veterinarians. Occasionally it is given by mouth for local antibacterial effects in the gastrointestinal tract.

Prevention

Patients should read the labels of all topical medications and avoid this agent as well as the following other antibacterials to which they may also have a reaction:

Bacitracin
Butirosin (Ambutyrosin)
Gentamicin (Garamycin)
Kanamycin

Paromomycin
Spectinomycin
Streptomycin
Tobramycin (Nebcin)

  Since some of these agents are present in prescription drugs (creams, ointments, pills, and injections), the patient should supply all health care providers with the above list.

May be duplicated for use in clinical practice. From Marks JG Jr, Elsner P, DeLeo VA: *Contact and occupational dermatology,* ed 3, St Louis, 2002, Mosby.

Neomycin and bacitracin sensitivity frequently occur concurrently in the same patient.

BIBLIOGRAPHY

Bjarnason B, Flosadóttir E: Patch testing with neomycin sulfate, *Contact Dermatitis* 43:295-302, 2000.

Cronin E: *Contact dermatitis,* London, 1980, Churchill Livingstone.

Gette MT, Marks JG, Maloney ME: Frequency of postoperative allergic contact dermatitis to topical antibiotics, *Arch Dermatol* 128:365-367, 1992.

Kimura M, Kawada A: Contact sensitivity induced by neomycin with cross-sensitivity to other aminoglycoside antibiotics, *Contact Dermatitis* 39:148-150, 1998.

Marks JG, Belsito DV, DeLeo VA et al: North American Contact Dermatitis Group standard tray patch test results: 1992 to 1994, *Am J Contact Dermat* 6:160-165, 1995.

Marks JG, Belsito DV, DeLeo VA et al: North American Contact Dermatitis Group standard tray patch test results: 1996 to 1998, *Arch Dermatol* 136:272-273, 2000.

Storrs F, Rosenthal LE, Adams RM et al: Prevalence and relevance of allergic reactions in patients tested in North America, *J Am Acad Dermatol* 20:1038-1044, 1989.

NICKEL

Definition

Nickel is a hard, strong, silver-white metal that resists corrosion and is used for electroplating and making alloys. Principal exposure is through costume (cheap) jewelry and other metal objects. Nickel is patch tested as 2.5% nickel sulfate in petrolatum in the United States. In Europe it is patch tested as 5% nickel sulfate in petrolatum. The T.R.U.E. Test contains 0.2 mg/cm^2 nickel sulfate in hydroxypropyl cellulose. The North American Contact Dermatitis Group found 14.2% of patch test clinic patients to be allergic to nickel, most being women or girls (Marks and others, 2000).

> **Nickel is the most common allergen in patch test clinics.**

Clinical Aspects

Delayed-type hypersensitivity to nickel is one of the most common allergies. At least 4.5% of the general population in Europe and 5.8% in the United States are allergic to this metal. Patch test clinics throughout the world have a high prevalence of nickel sensitivity, in the range of 15% with a significantly rising prevalence in some European countries approaching 30% to 40%. This is undoubtedly related to ear piercing. A study by Fischer and others (1984) in Sweden showed that all metal pins used for ear piercing released nickel in varying amounts, thus allowing exposure to the antigen. Not only are women and schoolgirls affected, but also men, now that ear piercing has become fashionable among them. Among schoolgirls with pierced ears, 13% were allergic to nickel. In contrast, only 1% without pierced ears exhibited nickel sensitivity. There is conflicting evidence as to how good a history is at predicting nickel sensitivity. Some studies have found a high correlation between a positive nickel patch test response and a history of jewelry sensitivity. In one study, 10 of 12 subjects developed dermatitis on the ears either shortly after ear piercing or after wearing low-quality pierced earrings. In other studies nickel sensitivity could not be reliably predicted from pretest historical information. Fewer than half of the subjects with positive patch test responses to nickel had a history of metal sensitivity. In addition, a significant number of subjects with a history of metal contact dermatitis had negative patch test responses to nickel. Therefore it is important to patch test all patients in whom nickel sensitivity is suspected.

The threshold for elicitation of allergic contact dermatitis to nickel varies widely among individuals. The lowest amount of nickel producing a reaction varied 250-fold, from 2.5% (5.2 mg) to 0.01% (0.47 mg). Nickel-leaching studies indicate that the amount of bioavailable nickel can exceed the provocation threshold from 1- to 93-fold, depending on the metal object and the leaching solution.

> **A history of jewelry sensitivity does not reliably predict the results of nickel patch tests.**

When compared with normal saline and synthetic sweat, plasma was the most effective solution for removing available nickel from earrings. This may explain the frequent induction of sensitization from ear piercing. To prevent the induction of nickel hypersensitivity, the European Union Nickel Directive has regulated metal objects having significant skin contact, such as earrings or buttons. Metal-containing alloys or nickel-containing surface coatings that release nickel in excess of 0.5 mg/cm^2 per week are banned. The dimethylglyoxime test is used to detect metal objects that release excessive amounts of nickel, but this test is not always sensitive enough to detect small amounts of nickel release that may cause or induce allergic contact dermatitis.

The dimethylglyoxime test is used to test metal objects for release of nickel.

Nickel sensitivity is usually acquired nonoccupationally from jewelry, especially from earrings and other metal objects on clothing. There are not many reports of occupationally induced nickel contact dermatitis. For example, female medical workers who have a lot of metal contact on the job have no greater allergy to nickel than the general female population does. Most of their nickel allergy was acquired before their working life.

The relationship of nickel oral ingestion to dermatitis is controversial. Nickel is found in food and water, but its relationship to the development of hand eczema following ingestion has been studied in double-blind clinical trials with mixed results. Some studies but not others show significant flare-ups of dermatitis after nickel ingestion. The amount of nickel content in food is quite variable, depending on the nickel content of the soil, the type of food, and the utensils used in preparation. These investigations used varying amounts of nickel in different study designs that led to varied results and interpretations. The consensus now, however, is that there is little enthusiasm for restriction of nickel in the diet of individuals with hand eczema. Likewise, the use of chelating agents such as disulfiram (Antabuse) has given conflicting results, and potential hepatotoxicity limits its use. Interestingly, one study indicated that schoolgirls who had oral metal appliances (braces) applied before the piercing of their ears had significantly less nickel allergy than did those who had not worn braces, thus indicating the induction of tolerance. The contribution of stainless-steel cooking utensils to nickel in the diet is negligible.

It is controversial whether oral ingestion of nickel can flare hand dermatitis.

Nickel sensitivity has caused concern with reference to implantation of orthopedic prostheses that are made with nickel alloys such as stainless steel or vitallium. Rarely, metal plates used to repair fractures have caused overlying allergic contact dermatitis. There is, however, no convincing evidence that modern plastic-to-metal joint prostheses containing nickel cause dermatitis or joint loosening in nickel-sensitive individuals. Furthermore, in patients with preexisting metal allergy, the implantation of cemented metal-to-plastic joint prosthesis is safe.

EXPOSURE LIST ▶ NICKEL

Synonyms and Other Names
Nickel is also known as niccolum sulfuricum.

Uses
Nickel is found in many metallic items either electroplated or as an alloy. The items often have a silvery appearance and include the following:

1. Costume jewelry (especially earrings, silver, and white gold)
2. Wearing apparel (snaps, zippers, and buttons)
3. Coins and keys
4. Tools, utensils, and instruments
5. Metal parts of furniture
6. Batteries
7. Machinery parts
8. Metal-cutting fluids and coolants
9. Nickel plating for alloys such as new silver, Chinese silver, and German silver
10. Mobile phones

Prevention
The most effective means of preventing nickel sensitization would be to reduce exposure to nickel from costume jewelry, particularly earrings. The European Union has banned metal objects, including earrings, necklaces, bracelets, rings, wristwatches, portions of garments, and eyeglass frames, that release nickel in excess of 0.5 mg/cm^2 per week. Although this regulation will not prevent all cases of nickel sensitization, it should make a significant difference.

To avoid nickel in earrings, stainless steel or surgical steel earrings are available from H & A Enterprises, 143-19 25th Ave., Whitestone, NY 11357; Roman Research, Inc., 33 Riverside Dr., Penbroke, Massachusetts 02359; or Avon Jewelry for Sensitive Skin (1-800-for-Avon). Medical-grade polycarbonate plastic earrings are made by Blomdahl AB, Box 2085, 30002 Halmstad, Sweden.

The *dimethylglyoxime test* is a rapid, easy method to determine the release of nickel from metal objects. Two drops each of a 1% solution of dimethylglyoxime in alcohol and a 10% solution of ammonium hydroxide in water are placed on a cotton swab that is then rubbed evenly against the test item for 30 seconds. The appearance of light pink to red on the swab indicates the release of enough nickel to cause allergic contact dermatitis. The dimethylglyoxime test (Allertest Ni) may be purchased from Allerderm Laboratories (P.O. Box 2070, Petaluma, CA 94953). Patients can purchase this test kit for self-use at home and at work to avoid contact with nickel-containing objects.

It seems unlikely that casual contact with keys, coins, and other articles such as doorknobs will be a problem without significant concomitant sweating and pressure. Covering handles of tools with plastic is helpful for workers such as hairdressers or textile workers who use such metal tools as scissors. Clioquinol ointment 3% appears to be an effective barrier to prevent nickel contact dermatitis.

EXPOSURE LIST ▶ *p*-PHENYLENEDIAMINE

Synonyms and Other Names

1,4-Benzenediamine	1,4-Phenylenediamine
Orsin	PPD
p-Aminoaniline	Rodol D
p-Phenylenediamine	Ursol D
p-Diaminobenzene	

Uses

p-Phenylenediamine (PPD) is the parent compound for permanent hair dyes and is a component of the following products and processes:
1. Cosmetics (permanent hair colors and some dark-colored cosmetics)
2. Primary intermediate in the production of azo-type dyes
3. Rarely, fur and leather dyes
4. Photographic developers
5. Rubber and plastics industry (antioxidants and accelerators)
6. Photocopying
7. Lithography (printing inks)
8. Oils, greases, and gasoline
9. Epoxy resin hardeners
10. Milk testing
11. Temporary tattoo

Prevention

Most cases of PPD sensitivity arise from the use of permanent hair dyes. Fully developed (oxidized), PPD dye is no longer an allergen, so hair or fur that has already been dyed is safe. For persons who want to continue dying their hair, semipermanent (not containing PPD) or temporary hair dyes are a good alternative. For a hairdresser, it is best to avoid dying clients' hair. Wearing of latex nitrile or 4-H gloves is helpful but interferes with manual dexterity. Besides avoiding PPD, patients may also be sensitive to the hair dye chemicals *p*-toluenediamine; *p*-aminodiphenylamine; 2,4-diaminoanisole; and *o*-aminophenol. Allergic individuals should be cautious about using permanent hair colors with these chemicals. Occasionally individuals with PPD sensitivity can react to other, similar chemicals including sulfa drugs, sulfonylurea diabetes medications, *p*-aminosalicylic acid, benzocaine and procaine anesthetics, and *p*-aminobenzoic acid sunscreens.

May be duplicated for use in clinical practice. From Marks JG Jr, Elsner P, DeLeo VA: *Contact and occupational dermatology,* ed 3, St Louis, 2002, Mosby.

---

can also be involved. Once the dye becomes fully oxidized, it is no longer allergenic; thus dyed hair does not cause dermatitis. This is particularly important, since hairdressers frequently cut dyed hair and sensitized individuals may want to wear dyed furs.

PPD must be tested as the free base, since phenylenediamine hydrochloride is not an adequate substitute for patch testing. Guinea pig maximization tests indicate that two oxidative products of PPD, *p*-benzoquinonine and Bandrowski's base, can also elicit positive patch test reactions. Cross-reactivity occurs between the hair dye related chemicals PPD, PTD, and *p*-aminophenol (PAP).

Fully oxidized *p*-phenylenediamine in dyed hair or fur does not cause allergic contact dermatitis.

Contact urticaria and contact leukoderma from PPD have rarely occurred.

BIBLIOGRAPHY

Adams RM, Maibach HI: A five-year study of cosmetic reactions, *J Am Acad Dermatol* 13:1062-1069, 1985.

Armstrong DKB, Jones AB, Smith HR et al: Occupational sensitization to *p*-phenylenediamine: a 17-year review, *Contact Dermatitis* 41:348-349, 1999.

de Groot AC, Bruynzeel DP, Bos JD et al: The allergens in cosmetics, *Arch Dermatol* 124:1525-1529, 1988.

Fisher AA, Dorman RI: The clinical significance of weak positive patch test reactions to certain allergens, *Cutis* 11:450-453, 1973.

Fisher AA, Pelzig A, Kanof NB: The persistence of allergic eczematous sensitivity and the cross-sensitivity pattern to paraphenylenediamine, *J Invest Dermatol* 30:9-12, 1958.

Fukunaga T, Kawagoe R, Hozumi H et al: Contact anaphylaxis due to para-phenylenediamine, *Contact Dermatitis* 35:185-186, 1996.

Le Coz CJ, Lefebvre C, Keller F et al: Allergic contact dermatitis caused by skin painting (pseudo-tattooing) with black henna, a mixture of henna and *p*-phenylenediamine and its derivatives, *Arch Dermatol* 136:1515-1517, 2000.

Marcoux D, Riboulet-Delmas G: Efficacy and safety of hair-coloring agents, *Am J Contact Dermat* 5:123-129, 1994.

Marks JG: Occupational skin disease in hairdressers, *Occup Med* 1:273-284, 1986.

Marks JG: The Accupatch: a new patch testing device, *Am J Contact Dermat* 2:98-101, 1991.

Marks, JG, Belsito DV, DeLeo VA et al: North American Contact Dermatitis Group standard tray patch test results: 1996 to 1998, *Arch Dermatol* 136:272-273, 2000.

Matkar NM: Natural and synthetic hair dyes: a solution for graying hair, *Cosmetics Toiletries* 115:77-86, 2000.

Mollgaard B, Hansen J, Kreilgaard B et al: Cross sensitization in guinea pigs between *p*-phenylenediamine and oxidation products thereof, *Contact Dermatitis* 23:274, 1990.

Rebandel P, Rudzki E: Occupational allergy to *p*-phenylenediamine in milk testers, *Contact Dermatitis* 33:138, 1995.

Reiss F, Fisher AA: Is hair dyed with para-phenylenediamine allergenic? *Arch Dermatol* 109:221-222, 1974.

Sidbury R, Storrs FJ: Pruritic eruption at the site of a temporary tattoo, *Am J Contact Dermat* 11:182-183, 2000.

Spengler J, Bracher M: Toxicological tests and health risk assessment of oxidative hair dye mixtures, *Cosmetics Toiletries* 105:67-76, 1990.

Storrs FJ, Taylor J, Jordan WP et al: Para-phenylenediamine dihydrochloride, *Contact Dermatitis* 5:126, 1979.

Xie Z, Hayakawa R, Sugiura M et al: Experimental study on skin sensitization potencies and cross-reactivities of hair-dye-related chemicals in guinea pigs, *Contact Dermatitis* 42:270-275, 2000.

p-tert-BUTYLPHENOL FORMALDEHYDE RESIN

Definition

p-tert-Butylphenol formaldehyde resin (PTBP formaldehyde resin) is one of a large group of synthetic polymers made by reacting formaldehyde with phenol or related alcohols to form network polymers. They are used primarily as adhesives and were the first synthetic polymers to be used commercially. The resin is tested at a 1% concentration in petrolatum or at 0.04 mg/cm² in hydroxypropyl cellulose in the T.R.U.E. Test. This antigen caused positive reactions in 1.8% of patch test clinic patients reported by the North American Contact Dermatitis Group (Marks and others, 2000).

Clinical Aspects

PTBP formaldehyde resin is one of a large group of formaldehyde-based phenol resins. PTBP or other phenols are reacted with formaldehyde to produce low-molecular-weight polymers called phenoplasts. The most frequent sensitizer in this group of plastics is PTBP formaldehyde resin. Unlike some of the other phenoplasts, it is used almost exclusively as a glue or an adhesive. This usage depends on its superior qualities of rapid adhesion, durability, and pliability. It cures slowly without additional hardeners at room temperature. The pliability and flexibility make it particularly useful in the bonding of shoe components and parts of watch straps, handbags, hats, and belts. For this purpose it is frequently combined with natural or synthetic rubber.

EXPOSURE LIST ▶ *p-tert*-BUTYLPHENOL FORMALDEHYDE RESIN

Synonyms and Other Names
Butylphen
4(1,1-Dimethylethyl)phenol
PTBP formaldehyde

Uses
p-tert-Butylphenol (PTBP) formaldehyde resin is used primarily as a glue in the following applications:
1. One-component glue or adhesive
2. Leather shoes, handbags, and watch straps
3. Plywood
4. Boxes
5. Insulation
6. Dental bonding
7. Automobiles
8. Motor oils
9. Disinfectants, deodorants, and insecticides
10. Inks and papers
11. Film developers
12. Diapers

Prevention
Patients allergic to PTBP formaldehyde resin are probably reacting to a liquid glue or adhesive. They could be using this product at work if they make leather goods, boxes, plywood, or insulation or if they work as dentists or dental technician/hygienists. Patients may be exposed at home if their hobbies include woodworking or ceramics. In either case these patients should change the type of adhesive they are using to one to which they are not allergic. If this is impossible, gloves should be worn for protection. Allergic patients may also be developing dermatitis at the site of contact with leather products glued with this agent, such as watch straps, shoes (see Box 5-2), or handbags, so dermatologists should test these suspected products for confirmation. Patients should be instructed to alert their dentist to their allergy, since this agent may be used in dentistry.

May be duplicated for use in clinical practice. From Marks JG Jr, Elsner P, DeLeo VA: *Contact and occupational dermatology,* ed 3, St Louis, 2002, Mosby.

> ***p-tert*-Butylphenol formaldehyde resins are used primarily as glues for leather products such as shoes, watch straps, and belts.**

The allergenic portion of the resin molecule is thought to be the phenol (PTBP), not formaldehyde. The polymerized resin produces a positive reaction when used for patch testing, but only the PTBP molecule is absolutely necessary in 50% to 90% of sensitized patients.

PTBP formaldehyde resin allergy may be occupationally related in cobblers and others who make leather goods with adhesives. Dental personnel, plywood and box makers, and insulation workers may also be exposed to the resin. The resin has also been used in automobile factories as a sealant.

The resin is used in glues available for home use in woodworking and ceramics, and approximately half of all sensitive individuals were sensitized in a nonoccupational setting. It occasionally produces dermatitis from its presence as an adhesive in shoes and other leather products.

PTBP formaldehyde resin sensitivity is frequently reported in individuals who are epoxy resin sensitive. Since the two resins are not chemically related, this cosensitivity is unexplained. PTBP has also been reported to induce chemical depigmentation.

PTBP is used infrequently as an oil demulsifier, film developer, disinfectant, deodorant, and insecticide, as well as in inks and papers.

BIBLIOGRAPHY
Cronin E: *Contact dermatitis,* London, 1980, Churchill Livingstone.
Malten KE: Occupational eczema due to paratertiary butylphenol in a shoe adhesive, *Dermatologica* 117:103-109, 1958.
Marks, JG, Belsito DV, DeLeo VA et al: North American Contact Dermatitis Group standard tray patch test results: 1996 to 1998, *Arch Dermatol* 136:272-273, 2000.
Shono M, Ezoe K, Kaniwa MA et al: Allergic contact dermatitis from paratertiary-butylphenol-formaldehyde resin (PTBP-FR) in athletic tape and leather adhesive, *Contact Dermatitis* 24:281-288, 1991.
Storrs F, Rosenthal LE, Adams RM et al: Prevalence and relevance of allergic reactions in patients tested in North America, *J Am Acad Dermatol* 20:1038-1044, 1989.
Zimerson E, Bruze M: Contact allergy to 5,5'-*di-tert*-butyl-2,2'-dihydroxy-(hydroxymethyl)-dibenzyl ethers, sensitizers in *p-tert*-butylphenol-formaldehyde resin, *Contact Dermatitis* 43:20-26, 2000.

PARABEN MIX
Definition
The parabens are alkyl esters of *p*-hydroxybenzoic acid. They are the most commonly used preservatives in cosmetics and are usually patch tested as a paraben mix (16% in petrolatum) containing 4% each of methyl, ethyl, propyl, and butyl parabens or 1 mg/cm^2 in polyvidone containing 0.162 mg each of methyl, ethyl, propyl, butyl, and benzyl parabens. The paraben mixtures are superior to the individual esters for patch testing, and *p*-hydroxybenzoic acid, the common paraben's metabolite in the skin, is not the hapten of parabens. The North American Contact Dermatitis Group found that 1.7% of their patients had positive patch test responses to the paraben mix (Marks and others, 2000).

> **Primin is the allergen in the houseplant *Primula obconica*.**

BIBLIOGRAPHY

Epstein E: *Primula* contact dermatitis: an easily overlooked diagnosis, *Cutis* 45:411-416, 1990.

Hausen BM, Heitsch H, Borrmann B, et al: Structure-activity relationships in allergic contact dermatitis. I. Studies on the influence of side-chain length with derivatives of primin, *Contact Dermatitis* 33:12-16, 1995.

Ingber A, Mennè T: Primin standard patch testing: 5 years' experience, *Contact Dermatitis* 23:15-19, 1990.

Tabar AI, Quirce S, Garcia E et al: Primula dermatitis: versatility in its clinical presentation and the advantages of patch tests with synthetic primin, *Contact Dermatitis* 30:47-48, 1994.

QUATERNIUM-15

Definition

Quaternium-15 is a broad-spectrum preservative found in many cosmetics and personal care products. A 2% concentration in petrolatum or 0.1 mg/cm^2 in hydroxypropyl cellulose gel was used in the standard tray. The North American Contact Dermatitis Group found that 9.0% of their patients had positive patch test reactions to quaternium-15 (Marks and others, 2000).

> **Quaternium-15 is the preservative that most frequently causes allergic contact dermatitis in the United States.**

Clinical Aspects

Quaternium-15 was the preservative causing the most contact allergy in the 5-year North American Contact Dermatitis Group study of cosmetic reactions. It has activity against bacteria, fungi, and molds and is particularly effective against *Pseudomonas aeruginosa* and *Pseudomonas cepacia*. Being water soluble, it is most effective in the aqueous phase of formulations, where it is needed. Its use concentration in cosmetics is generally between 0.02% and 0.3%.

Quaternium-15 is a member of the quaternary ammonium compounds that include benzalkonium chloride. As a group other than quaternium-15, the quaternary ammonium compounds tend to be infrequent sensitizers, but they are irritants that can make patch testing interpretation difficult. Quaternium-15 is also one of the formaldehyde-releasing preservatives that include imidazolidinyl urea, diazolidinyl urea, 2-bromo-2-nitropropane-1,3-diol, dimethylolmethyl (DMDM) hydantoin, and tris (hydroxymethyl) nitromethane. Although quaternium-15 does release small amounts of formaldehyde, not all patients who are allergic to quaternium-15 are allergic to formaldehyde and vice versa. The amount of formaldehyde released by quaternium-15 is less than the threshold reactivity in most formaldehyde-sensitive individuals. Thus many formaldehyde-sensitive individuals can use products containing quaternium-15 without developing allergic contact dermatitis. Patients who are sensitized to quaternium-15 may be allergic to quaternium-15 itself or to the formaldehyde released from this preservative. It has been shown, however, that patients presensitized to formaldehyde do develop dermatitis from lotions and creams containing quaternium-15.

EXPOSURE LIST ▷ **QUATERNIUM-15**

Synonyms and Other Names
1-(3-Chloroallyl)-3,5,7-triaza-1-azoniaadamantane chloride
Chloroallyl methenamine chloride
Azoniaadamantane chloride
cis-1-(3-Chloroallyl)3,5,7-triaza-1-azoniaadamantane chloride
Dowicil 75, 100, 200 (chemically similar)
Dowicil 200
Methenamine-3-chloroallylochloride
N-(3-Chloroallyl) hexaminium chloride
Preventol D 1

Uses
Quaternium-15 is a preservative that is found in many cosmetics and is used in industrial applications, as follows:
1. Cosmetics (creams, lotions, shampoos, and soaps)
2. Medicated creams, ointments, and lotions
3. Latex paints
4. Polishes and waxes
5. Jointing cements
6. Metalworking fluids
7. Adhesives
8. Construction materials
9. Paper or paperboard
10. Inks
11. Textile finishing solutions
12. Spinning emulsions
13. Photocopier toner

Prevention
The most common cause of allergic contact dermatitis from quaternium-15 is cosmetics preserved with this chemical. Careful label reading allows avoidance. Some individuals who are allergic to formaldehyde are also sensitive to quaternium-15, since quaternium-15 releases small amounts of formaldehyde. Quaternium-15–sensitive individuals may need to avoid cosmetics preserved with formaldehyde or formaldehyde-releasing agents, such as 2-bromo-2-nitropropane-1,3-diol, quaternium-15, imidazolidinyl urea, diazolidinyl urea, DMDM hydantoin, and tris (hydroxymethyl) nitromethane.

May be duplicated for use in clinical practice. From Marks JG Jr, Elsner P, DeLeo VA: *Contact and occupational dermatology,* ed 3, St Louis, 2002, Mosby.

The prevalence of sensitivity to quaternium-15 varies from one country to another. The Swiss Contact Dermatitis Research Group found only 1.0% of their patients to be allergic to quaternium-15, whereas 4.3% had positive reactions in the United Kingdom and 9.6% in the United States (Fransway, 1995).

Quaternium-15 has excellent preservative properties in formulations and is effective over a broad pH range of 4 to 10. It is a free-flowing powder that disperses and dissolves readily in the aqueous phase of formulations. Its compatibility with proteins and surfactants contributes to product stability. As a dried powder or a 10% solution, quaternium-15 is essentially nonirritating to the skin. Cosmetics with low concentrations of quaternium-15 are effectively preserved for 2 or more years.

CHAPTER 6

Preservatives and Vehicles

Preservatives ▬▬▬

Preservatives are used widely in cosmetics, pharmaceuticals, and industrial applications (e.g., in metalworking fluids) to prevent spoilage from bacterial and fungal overgrowth. Following fragrances, preservatives are the second most common cosmetic ingredient causing contact dermatitis. In metalworking fluids, preservatives are the most common cause of allergic contact dermatitis.

> **Preservatives are the second most common cause of cosmetic allergic contact dermatitis.**

The ideal preservative kills microorganisms under conditions of normal use but at the same time has no toxic effect on humans, such as allergic contact dermatitis. Despite hundreds of chemicals that have preservative action, only a limited number are used because of the safety and effectiveness of these compounds when placed in the final product.

The ideal preservative should have (1) broad antimicrobial activity, (2) effectiveness over a wide range of pH values, (3) effectiveness for the entire shelf life of the product, (4) antimicrobial activity in both oil and water vehicles, (5) compatibility with other ingredients, (6) nontoxic and nonirritating qualities, and (7) low cost. The most commonly used cosmetic preservatives are listed in Table 6-1. The numerous categories of preservatives are listed in Table 6-2.

In Table 6-3, the frequency of preservative use in cosmetic formulas and positive patch test responses are compared. An important group of preservatives, the

Table 6-1	**Frequency of Preservative Use in Cosmetic Formulations**		
Preservative	1980*	1990*	1993*
Parabens (methyl, propyl, butyl, ethyl)	13,786	16,107	15,020
Imidazolidinyl urea	1684	2749	2312
Butylated hydroxyanisole (BHA)	518	601	1669
Butylated hydroxytoluene (BHT)	404	551	1610
Methylchloroisothiazolinone/methylisothiazolinone	38	711	1042
Phenoxyethanol	25	375	929
DMDM hydantoin	79	550	747
Quaternium-15	1011	705	639
Diazolidinyl urea	0	280	466
2-Bromo-2-nitropropane-1, 3-diol	566	321	223
Formaldehyde	874	441	185

*Number of formulations that contain the preservative.

Table 6-2	Categories of Preservatives	
Alcohols		Organic compounds
Amides and amines		Paraben esters
Carbanilides		Phenol derivatives
Formaldehyde donors		Pyridine compounds
Inorganics		Quaternium compounds
Metal compounds		UV absorbers

Table 6-3 — Frequency of Preservative Use in Cosmetic Formulas and of Positive Patch Test Responses

Preservative	Number of Products With the Preservative (1996)*	Positive Patch Test Responses: 1996-1998 (%)†
Parabens (methyl, propyl, butyl, ethyl)	17,240	1.7
Imidazolidinyl urea	2498	2.5
DMDM hydantoin	955	2.6
Methylchloroisothiazolinone/ methylisothiazolinone	808	2.9
Quaternium-15	704	9.0
Diazolidinyl urea	690	2.9
2-Bromo-2-nitropropane-1, 3-diol	210	3.2
Formaldehyde	187	9.3
Methyldibromo glutaronitrile	57	2.7

*United States Food and Drug Administration Data in *J Cosmetics Toiletries,* 1997.
†North American Contact Dermatitis Group (Marks and others, 2000).

formaldehyde donors, are listed in Table 6-4. The International Nomenclature Cosmetic Ingredient (INCI) names, and brand names of preservatives are listed in Table 6-5. The INCI name is on the cosmetic ingredient label and is the name the patient must know to avoid contact dermatitis.

The patient must know the INCI (International Nomenclature Cosmetic Ingredient) name to avoid the allergen in cosmetics.

The reader is referred to Chapter 5 for review of the preservatives found on the standard series: formaldehyde, imidazolidinyl urea, methylchloroisothiazolinone/methylisothiazolinone, parabens, quaternium-15, and thimerosal.

Table 6-4
Formaldehyde Donors

5-Bromo-5-nitro-1, 3-dioxane	Hydantoin
2-Bromo-2-nitropropane-1, 3-diol	Imidazolidinyl urea
Diazolidinyl urea	MDM hydantoin
DMDM hydantoin	p-formaldehyde
DMHP	Quaternium-15
Formaldehyde solution	Tris (hydroxymethyl) nitromethane
Glutaral (glutaraldehyde)	

Table 6-5
International Nomenclature Cosmetic Ingredient (INCI) Names and Brand Names for Preservatives

INCI Name	Brand or Generic Name
Methylchloroisothiazolinone/methylisothiazolinone	Kathon CG
Quaternium-15	Dowicil 200
2-Bromo-2-nitropropane-1, 3-diol	Bronopol
Imidazolidinyl urea	Germall 115
Diazolidinyl urea	Germall II
DMDM hydantoin	Glydant

BIBLIOGRAPHY

Andersen KE, Rycroft RJG: Recommended patch test concentrations for preservatives, biocides, and antimicrobials, *Contact Dermatitis* 25:1-18, 1991.

Barker MO: Cosmetic preservation issues, *Am J Contact Dermat* 4:182-184, 1993.

Marks JG, Belsito DV, DeLeo VA, et al: North American Contact Dermatitis Group standard tray patch test results, 1996 to 1998, *Arch Dermatol* 136:272-273, 2000.

Marks JG, Belsito DV, DeLeo VA, et al: North American Contact Dermatitis Group standard tray patch test results: 1992 to 1994, *Am J Contact Dermat* 6:160-165, 1995.

Mustcatiello MJ: CTFA's preservation guidelines: a historical perspective and review, *Cosmetics Toiletries* 108:53-59, 1993.

Skinner SL, Marks JG: Allergic contact dermatitis to preservatives in topical medicaments, *Am J Contact Dermat* 9:199-201, 1998.

Steinberg DC: Frequency of use of preservatives: a review of the preservatives reported as used in products sold in the United States, *Cosmetics Toiletries* 112:57-65, 1997.

Steinberg DC: Cosmetic preservation: current international trends, *Cosmetics Toiletries* 107:77-82, 1992.

BENZYL ALCOHOL
Definition

Benzyl alcohol is an aromatic organic alcohol that is a preservative, a solvent, a local anesthetic, and a fragrance. It is patch tested as a 1% concentration in petrolatum. It is a relatively uncommon sensitizer, and 0.2 % to 1% of patients attending patch test clinics have a positive reaction to benzyl alcohol.

| EXPOSURE LIST | BENZYL ALCOHOL |

Synonyms or Other Names

Benzenemethanol   Phenylmethanol
Phenylcarbinol   α-Hydroxytoluene

Uses

Benzyl alcohol is a preservative, solvent, and fragrance used in cosmetics, medicated products, and industry. It has the following applications:

1. Cosmetics including fragrances
2. Flavors
3. Medications
4. Bean slackers, photo developers, inks, adhesives, flooring materials, cleaning agents, cutting oils
5. Solvent for gelatin, casein, cellulose acetate, shellac
6. Microscopy imbedding material
7. Ear mold impression material

Prevention

Cosmetics, medicines, and industrial products that contain benzyl alcohol must be avoided. This can be accomplished by reading cosmetic labels, package inserts, and material safety data sheets.

May be duplicated for use in clinical practice. From Marks JG Jr, Elsner P, DeLeo VA: *Contact and occupational dermatology,* ed 3, St Louis, 2002, Mosby.

Clinical Aspects

Benzyl alcohol is extensively used in fragrances, flavors, photography, hair dyes, plastics, inks, and pharmaceuticals. It is added to allergen extracts and injectable solutions as a preservative and is a constituent of jasmine, hyacinth, ylang-ylang oils, balsams of Peru and Tolu, and storax. It has a faint aromatic odor with a sharp burning taste. It is produced on a large scale by the action of sodium or potassium carbonate on benzyl chloride.

Benzyl alcohol has widespread use in cosmetics, medicines, and industrial applications. Cases of allergic contact dermatitis from benzyl alcohol have been reported from fragrances, cutting oil deodorant, flavored beverages, epoxy adhesives, topical and injectable medications, and hearing aid impression material.

> **Benzyl alcohol is a preservative, solvent, and fragrance material used in many products. It is an uncommon cause of allergic contact dermatitis.**

BIBLIOGRAPHY

Podda M, Zollner T, Grundmann-Kollmann M et al: Allergic contact dermatitis from benzyl alcohol during topical antimycotic treatment, *Contact Dermatitis* 41:302-303, 1999.

Shaw DW: Allergic contact dermatitis to benzyl alcohol in a hearing aid impression material, *Am J Contact Dermat* 10:228-232, 1999.

| **EXPOSURE LIST** | **2-BROMO-2-NITROPROPANE-1,3-DIOL** |

Synonyms or Other Names

Bronopol   1,3-Propanediol-2-bromo-2-nitro
Lexgard bronopol   Myacide BT
Onyxide 500

Uses

Bronopol is a preservative that is used in cosmetic formulations and other applications that require preservation, including the following:

1. Cosmetics (makeup, hair conditioners, shampoos, mascara, cleansing lotions, and moisturizers)
2. Medicated products
3. Milk sampling
4. Simulated silage
5. Household products (fabric conditioners and washing detergents)
6. Paints
7. Textiles
8. Hide processing
9. Cooling towers
10. Humidifiers
11. Adhesives
12. Paper
13. Pesticides

Prevention

Avoidance of 2-bromo-2-nitropropane-1,3-diol is accomplished by not using cosmetics or other products that contain this chemical as its preservative. It should be noted that some patients who are allergic to formaldehyde or other formaldehyde-releasing preservatives may not be able to tolerate 2-bromo-2-nitropropane-1,3-diol because it can also release small amounts of formaldehyde. On the other hand, a number of patients who are sensitive to 2-bromo-2-nitropropane-1,3-diol are not allergic to formaldehyde or formaldehyde-releasing preservatives. Inspection of the materials safety data sheets identifies industrial sources of exposure.

May be duplicated for use in clinical practice. From Marks JG Jr, Elsner P, DeLeo VA: *Contact and occupational dermatology*, ed 3, St Louis, 2002, Mosby.

2-BROMO-2-NITROPROPANE-1,3-DIOL

Definition

2-Bromo-2-nitropropane-1,3-diol (bronopol) is a preservative used in cosmetics, topical medicaments, and industry. It is patch tested at a 0.5% concentration in petrolatum. The North American Contact Dermatitis Group found 3.2% of its patients to be allergic to this biocide (Marks and others, 2000).

Clinical Aspects

2-Bromo-2-nitropropane-1,3-diol is a broad-spectrum preservative that is especially active against the gram-negative bacterium *Pseudomonas aeruginosa.* Two hundred ten cosmetic formulations were reported to use this biocide in the United States in 1996, but its use has declined in the past decade. Cosmetic preparations contain bronopol in most cases in concentrations of 0.01% to 0.02%. The Cosmetic Ingredient Review panel concluded that concentrations up to and including 0.1% were safe except when its action with amines or amides could result in the formation of nitrosamines or nitrosamides. When the concentration is raised to 1% or greater, it may be a significant irritant. Bronopol is a formaldehyde-releasing biocide with an emulsion that contains 0.02% bronopol releasing up to 15 ppm formaldehyde. Thus formaldehyde-sensitive patients may react to a product containing bronopol. Concomitant sensitization to bronopol and formaldehyde is found in about a third of patch test clinic patients. Storrs and Bell (1983) reported seven patients in whom allergic contact dermatitis developed after using a bronopol-preserved moisturizing cream on inflamed skin. None of their patients were allergic to formaldehyde or other formaldehyde-releasing preservatives. Their other patients, however, who were sensitized to bronopol in other cosmetics, had previously been sensitive to formaldehyde and to other formaldehyde-releasing preservatives.

> **2-Bromo-2-nitropropane-1,3-diol (bronopol) is a formaldehyde releaser and may cause contact dermatitis in formaldehyde-sensitive or formaldehyde-releasing preservative–sensitive individuals.**

BIBLIOGRAPHY

Cosmetic Ingredient Review: Addendum to the final report on the safety assessment of 2-bromo-2-nitropropane-1,3-diol, *J Am Coll Toxicol* 3:139-155, 1984.

Croshaw B, Holland VR: Chemical preservatives: use of bronopol as a cosmetic preservative. In Kabara JJ, editor: *Cosmetic and drug preservation: principles and practice,* New York, 1984, Marcel Dekker.

Fisher AA: Cosmetic dermatitis: reactions to some commonly used preservatives, *Cutis* 26:136-137, 144-142, 147-148, 1980.

Frosch PJ, White IR, Rycroft RJG et al: Contact allergy to bronopol, *Contact Dermatitis* 22:24-26, 1990.

Gruening R: Bromo-organic preservatives, *Cosmetics Toiletries* 114:63-71, 1999.

Marks JG, Belsito DV, DeLeo VA et al: North American Contact Dermatitis Group standard tray patch test results: 1996 to 1998, *Arch Dermatol* 136:272-273, 2000.

Storrs FJ, Bell DE: Allergic contact dermatitis to 2-bromo-2-nitropropane-1,3-diol in hydrophilic ointment, *J Am Acad Dermatol* 8:157-170, 1983.

BUTYLATED HYDROXYANISOLE AND BUTYLATED HYDROXYTOLUENE (BHA AND BHT)

Definition

The antioxidants butylated hydroxyanisole (BHA) and butylated hydroxytoluene (BHT) are commonly used in cosmetics and foods. They are tested at 5% concentration in petrolatum. Allergic contact dermatitis to these chemicals is rare. The North American Contact Dermatitis Group found 0.2% and 0.1% of their contact dermatitis clinic patients had positive reactions to BHA and BHT, respectively (Marks and others, 1995).

Clinical Aspects

BHA and BHT are antioxidants used in foods, cosmetics, medicaments, and industry. BHA and BHT were the third and fourth most common preservatives, respectively, used in cosmetic formulations reported to the United States Food and Drug Administration in 1993. The addition of antioxidants such as BHA and BHT prevent undesirable changes (1) in color such as the browning of fresh apples and peaches when exposed to air and (2) in flavor such as the rancid taste and odor that develops in fats, oil, mayonnaise, and lard. Up to 200 ppm of BHA and BHT may be used for food preservation.

Roed-Petersen and Hjorth (1976) reported two sensitized women who had hand eczema from either BHT or BHA. When they avoided topical medicaments and eating foods containing these antioxidants, their eczema cleared. Both patients had flare-ups of the hand eczema after oral provocation tests with small amounts of BHA or BHT. Fisher reported a cook with chronic hand eczema and perioral dermatitis from mayonnaise preserved with BHA; this person had positive patch test responses to the mayonnaise and 2% BHA (Rietschel and Fowler, 1995). When the cook avoided the incriminated mayonnaise, his hands and mouth cleared. Contact urticaria and intensification of rhinitis and asthma have also been reported after the ingestion of BHA and BHT.

BHA and BHT are rare sensitizers. These antioxidants are found in numerous cosmetics, medicaments, and foods and in industry.

EXPOSURE LIST ▷ BHA AND BHT

Synonyms and Other Names

BHA
  Butylated hydroxyanisole
  2-tert-Butyl-4-methoxyphenol
  Embanox
  4-Methoxy-2-tert-butylphenol
  Nipantiox 1-F
  Phenol (1,1-dimethylethyl)-4-methoxy
  Sustane 1-F
  Tenox
  Vyox

BHT
  Annulex BHT
  2,6-Bis(1,1-dimethylethyl)-4-methylphenol
  Butylated hydroxytoluene
  Catalin CAO-3
  2,6-Di-tert-butyl-cresol
  DBPC
  Embanox BHT
  Hydagen DEO
  Ionol
  4-Methyl-2,6-di-tert-butyl-phenol
  Tenox BHT
  Topanol OC and O

Uses

BHA and BHT are used as preservatives (antioxidants) in foods, cosmetics, and industry and have the following applications:
  1. Cosmetics
  2. Foods (beverages, gum, ice cream, fruits, and cereals)
  3. Medicated cream and gels
  4. Animal feeds
  5. Petroleum products
  6. Jet fuels
  7. Rubber
  8. Plastics
  9. Paints
  10. Glues

Prevention

Reading labels and material safety data sheets is necessary to avoid the widespread presence of these chemicals.

BIBLIOGRAPHY

Flyvholm M, Mennè T: Sensitizing risk of butylated hydroxytoluene based on exposure and effect data, *Contact Dermatitis* 23:341-345, 1990.

Marks JG, Belsito DV, DeLeo VA et al: North American Contact Dermatitis Group standard tray patch test results: 1992 to 1994, *Am J Contact Dermat* 6:160-165, 1995.

Meneghini CL, Rantuccio F, Lomuto M: Additives, vehicles, and active drugs of topical medicaments as causes of delayed-type allergic dermatitis, *Dermatologica* 143:137, 1971.

Rietschel RL, Fowler JF: *Fisher's contact dermatitis,* ed 4, Baltimore, 1995, Williams & Wilkins.

Roed-Petersen J, Hjorth N: Contact dermatitis from antioxidants: hidden sensitizers in topical medications and foods, *Br J Dermatol* 94:233-241, 1976.

Turner TW: Dermatitis from butylated hydroxyanisole, *Contact Dermatitis* 3:282, 1977.

CHLORINATED BIOCIDES

Chlorinated water, sodium hypochlorite, chloramine-T, and chlorhexidine (Arlacide) are rare sensitizers. The latter two compounds have replaced quaternary ammonium compounds as disinfectant skin cleansers, antiseptic mouth rinses, and for the treatment of burns. One study of patients with leg ulcers, however, found that up to 13% may be sensitized to chlorhexidine (Knudsen and Avnstorp, 1991). The North American Contact Dermatitis Group patch tests with chlorhexidine gluconate, 1% aqueous (Marks and others, 1995).

BIBLIOGRAPHY

Knudsen BB, Avnstorp C: Chlorhexidine gluconate and acetate in patch testing, *Contact Dermatitis* 24:45-49, 1991.

Marks JG, Belsito DV, DeLeo VA et al: North American Contact Dermatitis Group standard tray patch test results: 1992 to 1994, *Am J Contact Dermat* 6:160-165, 1995.

p-CHLORO-*m*-CRESOL

Definition

p-Chloro-*m*-cresol is a substituted phenol that is used more commonly in medicaments than in cosmetics because of its bad smell. It is patch tested as a 1% concentration in petrolatum. The North American Contact Dermatitis Group found 0.4% of their patch test clinic patients to be sensitive to this biocide (Marks and others, 1995).

Clinical Aspects

p-Chloro-*m*-cresol is a strong sensitizer in the guinea pig maximization test. This is in direct contrast to clinical experience in which *p*-chloro-*m*-cresol is a rare sensitizer, despite being widely used as a preservative in pharmaceutical products and in industry. Topical corticosteroids containing *p*-chloro-*m*-cresol, particularly betamethasone cream preparations, have been the most frequently reported cause of allergic contact dermatitis from this preservative.

> **Some corticosteroid creams are preserved with *p*-chloro-*m*-cresol, particularly betamethasone.**

EXPOSURE LIST ▶ *p*-CHLORO-*m*-CRESOL

Synonyms and Other Names

4-Chloro-3-methylphenol

Chlorocresol

Ottafect

Parachlorometacresol

PCMC

Phenol, 4-chloro-3-methyl

Preventol CMK

Uses

p-Chloro-*m*-cresol is a preservative that is widely used in medicated products, cosmetics, and industry and has the following applications:

1. Medicated products (corticosteroid creams)
2. Cosmetics (shampoos and baby cosmetics)
3. Topical antiseptics and disinfectants
4. Adhesives and glues
5. Inks, paints, and varnishes
6. Textile finishes
7. Packing materials
8. Tanning agents
9. Metalworking fluids

Prevention

Topical preparations containing this preservative, particularly corticosteroid creams, should be avoided. The drug package insert and cosmetic label should be read carefully. The materials safety data sheets should be helpful in locating industrial sources of exposure. Preparations containing chloroxylenol (*p*-chloro-*m*-xylenol [PCMX]) should also be avoided, since there is cross-reactivity with this similar chemical preservative.

May be duplicated for use in clinical practice. From Marks JG Jr, Elsner P, DeLeo VA: *Contact and occupational dermatology,* ed 3, St Louis, 2002, Mosby.

BIBLIOGRAPHY

Andersen KE, Hamann K: How sensitizing is chlorocresol? Allergy test in guinea pigs vs. the clinical experience, *Contact Dermatitis* 11:11-20, 1984.

Burry JN, Kirk J, Reid JG et al: Chlorocresol sensitivity, *Contact Dermatitis* 1:41-42, 1975.

Dooms-Goossens A, Degreef H, Van Hee J et al: Chlorocresol and chloracetamide: allergens in medications, glues and cosmetics, *Contact Dermatitis* 7:51-52, 1981.

Marks JG, Belsito DV, DeLeo VA et al: North American Contact Dermatitis Group standard tray patch test results: 1992 to 1994, *Am J Contact Dermat* 6:160-165, 1995.

CHLOROXYLENOL

Definition

Chloroxylenol is a substituted phenolic biocide that is used predominantly in medications and household products with disinfectant properties. It is patch tested at 1% concentration in petrolatum. The North American Contact Dermatitis Group found 1.0% of their patients to be allergic to this chemical (Marks and others, 2000).

Clinical Aspects

Chloroxylenol is a halogenated phenolic disinfectant that has greater antimicrobial activity than *p*-chloro-*m*-cresol and is 60 times more potent than phenol. When

---

EXPOSURE LIST ▷ **CHLOROXYLENOL**

Synonyms and Other Names

Benzytol
4-Chloro-3,5-dimethylphenol
4-Chloro-3,5-xylenol
Dettol
Husept extra

Nipacide PX
Ottasept
p-Chloro-*m*-xylenol
Parachlorometaxylenol
PCMX

Uses

1. Cosmetics (soaps and hair conditioners)
2. Over-the-counter topical medications
3. Household and hospital disinfectants
4. Electrocardiogram paste
5. Carbolated petroleum jelly
6. Urinary antiseptics

Prevention

Products that contain chloroxylenol must be avoided by reviewing the ingredients listed on the package, package insert, or material safety data sheets. *p*-Chloro-*m*-cresol should also be avoided, since patients sensitive to chloroxylenol may also react to *p*-chloro-*m*-cresol.

May be duplicated for use in clinical practice. From Marks JG Jr, Elsner P, DeLeo VA: *Contact and occupational dermatology*, ed 3, St Louis, 2002, Mosby.

---

hexachlorophene was withdrawn from nonprescription drugs in the United States, chloroxylenol was frequently substituted for it. Reports of allergic contact dermatitis are infrequent but have occurred after the use of medicated petroleum jelly (Vaseline) and electrocardiogram paste. Chloroxylenol is a popular household and hospital disinfectant, and the authors have seen housekeepers who developed allergic contact dermatitis from this preservative in liquid soaps. A number of patients who are sensitive to chloroxylenol also show sensitivity to *p*-chloro-*m*-cresol. The antigenic determinant of these compounds requires the presence of a chloride atom on the para position of the phenol ring.

> **Chloroxylenol is a popular disinfectant. It cross-reacts with *p*-chloro-*m*-cresol.**

BIBLIOGRAPHY

Marks JG, Belsito DV, DeLeo VA et al: North American Contact Dermatitis Group standard tray patch test results: 1996 to 1998, *Arch Dermatol* 136:272-273, 2000.

Mowad C: Chloroxylenol causing hand dermatitis in a plumber, *Am J Contact Dermat* 9:128-129, 1998.

Storrs FJ: Para-chloro-meta-xylenol allergic contact dermatitis in 7 individuals, *Contact Dermatitis* 1:211-213, 1975.

Zemtsov A, Guccione J, Cameron GS, Mattioli F: Evaluation of antigenic determinant in chlorocresol and chloroxylenol contact dermatitis by patch testing with chemically related substances, *Am J Contact Dermat* 5:19-21, 1994.

| EXPOSURE LIST | DIAZOLIDINYL UREA |

Synonyms and Other Names
Germall II
N,N^I-Bis (hydroxymethyl) urea
N-(hydroxymethyl)-N-(1,3-dihydroxymethyl-2,5-dioxo-4-imidazolidinyl)-N^I-(hydroxymethyl) urea
Germaben II (mixture)

Uses
Diazolidinyl urea is used as a preservative in cosmetics such as hair gels, creams, and body lotions. It may also be found in mediated creams and gels.

Prevention
Patients who are allergic to diazolidinyl urea should avoid cosmetics that contain this chemical. In addition, some diazolidinyl urea–sensitive patients may also be allergic to formaldehyde and formaldehyde-releasing preservatives such as imidazolidinyli urea, 2-bromo-2-nitropropane-1,3-diol, quaternium-15, DMDM hydantoin, and tris (hydroxymethyl) nitromethane.

May be duplicated for use in clinical practice. From Marks JG Jr, Elsner P, DeLeo VA: *Contact and occupational dermatology*, ed 3, St Louis, 2002, Mosby.

DIAZOLIDINYL UREA

Definition

Diazolidinyl urea is the newest and most active member of the imidazolidinyl urea family of preservatives. It is patch tested at a 1% concentration in water. The North American Contact Dermatitis Group found 3.7% of their patients to be allergic to this chemical (Marks and others, 2000).

Clinical Aspects

Diazolidinyl urea was introduced into cosmetics in the early 1980s at recommended concentrations of 0.1% to 0.5% and is approved for use in the United States and Europe, but not Japan. In 1996, 690 cosmetic products reported to the United States Food and Drug Administration contained diazolidinyl urea. It has a wider antimicrobial spectrum than imidazolidinyl urea and is particularly effective against *Pseudomonas* species and other gram-negative bacteria. It is used in combination with parabens or other antifungal preservatives. A solution of 0.3% diazolidinyl urea, 0.11% methyl paraben, and 0.03% propyl paraben is marketed under the trade name Germaben II.

> **Diazolidinyl urea is a formaldehyde-releasing preservative and may be more sensitizing than imidazolidinyl urea, with which it sometimes cross-reacts.**

In 1985, Kantor and others reported the first case of allergic contact dermatitis from diazolidinyl urea contained in a hair gel. de Groot and others (1988) more recently reported four cases of contact allergy to this biocide which was used in a "hypoallergenic" brand of cosmetics in the Netherlands. A drawback of

EXPOSURE LIST ▶	METHYLDIBROMO GLUTARONITRILE PHENOXYETHANOL

Synonyms and Other Names

2-Bromo-2(bromomethyl) glutaronitrile   Euxyl K-400
2-Bromo-2-(bromomethyl) pentanedinitrile   Merquat 2200
1,2-Dibromo-2,4-dicyanobutane   2-Phenoxyethanol
Dibromodicyanobutane   Tektamer 38

Uses

1. Cosmetics
2. Topical medicines
3. Metalworking fluids
4. Latex paints
5. Adhesives and glues
6. Wood preservatives
7. Seed disinfectants
8. Paper and moist toilet paper
9. Color photograph solutions
10. Ultrasonic gels
11. Cleansers and detergents
12. Sunscreen

Prevention

Products that contain methyldibromo glutaronitrile phenoxyethanol can be avoided by reading cosmetic labels, package inserts in topical medicines, and workplace material safety data sheets.

_____

May be duplicated for use in clinical practice. From Marks JG Jr, Elsner P, DeLeo VA: *Contact and occupational dermatology,* ed 3, St Louis, 2002, Mosby.

of contact allergy to methyldibromo glutaronitrile phenoxyethanol's active ingredients. A 43-year-old German patient, using a wrinkle-removing lotion on the face and neck, developed allergic contact dermatitis to this preservative mixture. Methyldibromo glutaronitrile (1,2-dibromo-2,4-dicyanobutane [Tektamer 38]) caused contact dermatitis in a 28-year-old maintenance mechanic from paste-glue that was used to fasten commercial labels to jars of baby food. Phenoxyethanol was reported to cause allergic contact dermatitis in a 53-year-old male office worker after exposure to an aqueous cream that was used as a soap substitute. Allergic contact dermatitis to the mixture has been reported from a number of products, including ultrasonic gel, cucumber eye gel, cosmetic creams, and moist toilet papers. The sensitization rates to this preservative mixture in European contact dermatitis clinics range from 0.5% to 2.8%.

> **Methyldibromo glutaronitrile phenoxyethanol is a preservative mixture found in cosmetics and personal care products. The main allergen in this mixture is methyldibromo glutaronitrile (1,2-dibromo-2,4-dicyanobutane).**

Methyldibromo glutaronitrile is the main allergen in this mixture, with phenoxyethanol having very little sensitizing potency. The Cosmetic Ingredient Review expert panel concluded that methyldibromo glutaronitrile is safe as used in rinse-off products (concentrations in cosmetic formulations range from 0.0075% to 0.06%) and safe in concentrations up to 0.025% in leave-on products. Although methyldibromo glutaronitrile phenoxyethanol is available commercially for patch testing at 0.5% in petrolatum, a 2% concentration may be preferable and some investigators use a 2.5% concentration; however, the latter concentration may cause irritant reactions. Other investigators use methyldibromo glutaronitrile alone at 0.3% in petrolatum.

BIBLIOGRAPHY

Bruze M, Gruverber B, Agrup G: Sensitization studies in the guinea pig with the active ingredients of Euxyl K-400, *Contact Dermatitis* 18:37-39, 1988.

Corazza M, Mantovani L, Roveggio C, Virgili A: Frequency of sensitization to Euxyl K-400 in 889 cases, *Contact Dermatitis* 28:298-299, 1993.

de Groot AC, Weyland JW: Contact allergy to methyldibromoglutaronitrile in the cosmetics preservative Euxyl K-400, *Am J Contact Dermat* 2:31-32, 1991.

Erdmann SM, Sachs B, Merk HF: Allergic contact dermatitis due to methyldibromo glutaronitrile in Euxyl K-400 in an ultrasonic gel, *Contact Dermatitis* 44:39-40, 2001.

Fernàndez E, Navarro JA, Del Pozo L, Fernàdez De Corrès L: Allergic contact dermatitis due to dibromodicyanobutane in cosmetics, *Contact Dermatitis* 109-110, 1995.

Gebhart M, Stuhlert A, Knopf B: Allergic contact dermatitis due to Euxyl K-400 in an ultrasonic gel, *Contact Dermatitis* 29:272, 1993.

Guimaraens D, Hernández MI, Gonzalez MA et al: Contact allergy to Euxyl K-400 in consecutively patch-tested patients, *Contact Dermatitis* 43:55-56, 2000.

Hausen BM: The sensitizing potency of Euxyl K-400 and its components 1,2-dibromo-2, 4-dicyanobutane and 2-phenoxyethanol, *Contact Dermatitis* 28:149-153, 1993.

Jackson JM, Fowler JF: Methyldibromoglutaronitrile (Euxyl K-400): a new and important sensitizer in the United States? *J Am Acad Dermatol* 38:934-937, 1998.

Lovell CR, White IR, Boyle J: Contact dermatitis from phenoxyethanol in aqueous cream BP, *Contact Dermatitis* 11:187, 1984.

Marks JG, Belsito DV, DeLeo VA et al: North American Contact Dermatitis Group standard tray patch test results: 1996 to 1998, *Arch Dermatol* 136:272-273, 2000.

Mathias CGT: Contact dermatitis to a new biocide (Textamer 38) used in a paste glue formulation, *Contact Dermatitis* 9:418-435, 1983.

McFadden JP, Ross JS, Jones AB et al: Increased rate of patch test reactivity to methyldibromo glutaronitrile, *Contact Dermatitis* 42:54-55, 2000.

O'Donnell BF, Foulds IS: Contact dermatitis due to dibromodicyanobutane in cucumber eye gel, *Contact Dermatitis* 29:99-100, 1993.

Ross JS, Cronin E, White IR, Rycroft RJG: Contact dermatitis from Euxyl K-400 in cucumber eye gel, *Contact Dermatitis* 26:60, 1992.

Senff H, Exner M, Gortz J, Goos M: Allergic contact dermatitis from Euxyl K-400, *Contact Dermatitis* 20:381, 1989.

Torres V, Soares AP: Contact allergy to dibromodicyanobutane in a cosmetic cream, *Contact Dermatitis* 27:114-115, 1992.

Tosti A, Guerra L, Bardazzi F, Gasparri F: Euxyl K-400: a new sensitizer in cosmetics, *Contact Dermatitis* 25:89-93, 1991.

Tosti A, Vincenzi C, Trevisi P, Guerra L: Euxyl K-400: incidence of sensitization, patch test concentration, and vehicle, *Contact Dermatitis* 33:193-195, 1995.

BIBLIOGRAPHY

Angelini G, Rigano L, Foti C et al: Contact allergy to impurities in surfactants: amount, chemical structure, and carrier effect in reactions to 3-dimethylaminopropylamine, *Contact Dermatitis* 34:248-252, 1996.

Angelini G, Foti C, Rigano L, Vena GA: 3-Dimethylaminopropylamine: a key substance in contact allergy to cocamidopropylbetaine? *Contact Dermatitis* 32:96-99, 1995.

Cosmetic Ingredient Review Expert Panel: Final Report on the Safety Assessment of Cocamidopropyl Betaine, *J Am Coll Toxicol* 10:33-52, 1991.

de Groot AC, van der Walle HB, Weyland JW: Contact allergy to cocamidopropyl betaine, *Contact Dermatitis* 33:419-422, 1995.

Fartasch M, Diepgen TL, Kuhn M et al: Provocative use tests in CAPB-allergic subjects with CAPB-containing product, *Contact Dermatitis* 41:30-34, 1999.

Fowler JF, Fowler LM, Hunter JE: Allergy to cocamidopropyl betaine may be due to amidomine: a patch test and product use test study, *Contact Dermatitis* 37:276-281, 1997.

Korting HC, Parsch EM, Enders F, Przybilla B: Allergic contact dermatitis to cocamidopropyl betaine in shampoo, *J Am Acad Dermatol* 27:1013-1015, 1992.

Pigatoo PD, Bigardi AS, Cusano F: Contact dermatitis to cocamidopropylbetaine is caused by residual amines: relevance, clinical characteristics, and review of the literature, *Am J Contact Dermat* 6:13-16, 1995.

OLEAMIDOPROPYL DIMETHYLAMINE

Oleamidopropyl dimethylamine is an amide-amine cationic emulsifier that was found to be a sensitizer in a body lotion for babies that women were applying on their faces. It is patch tested as a 0.4% concentration in an aqueous solution. Cross-reactions occur to related amide-amine–type cationic surfactants such as ricinoleamidopropyl dimethylamine lactate and tallowamidopropyl dimethylamine.

Synonyms and other names for this compound include diamethylaminopropyl oleamide, Lexamine 0-13, Mazeen OA, Schercodine O, and *N*-(3-dimethylaminopropyl)-9-octadecenamide.

BIBLIOGRAPHY

de Groot AC: *Adverse reactions to cosmetics,* thesis, The Netherlands, 1988, State University of Groningen.

de Groot AC, Bruynzeel DP, Bos JD et al: The allergens in cosmetics, *Arch Dermatol* 124:1525-1529, 1988.

Tosti A, Guerra AL, Morelli R et al: Prevalence and sources of sensitization to emulsifiers: a clinical study, *Contact Dermatitis* 23:68-72, 1990.

PROPYL GALLATE
Definition

Propyl gallate is the aromatic ester of propyl alcohol and gallic acid. It is an antioxidant used in cosmetic products, particularly lipsticks. It is one of a family of gallate esters including octyl and dodecyl gallate. Propyl gallate is patch tested at a concentration of 1% in petrolatum.

EXPOSURE LIST ▶ **PROPYL GALLATE**

Synonyms and Other Names

Benzoic acid, 3,4,5-trihydroxy-propyl ester
Embanox
Gallic acid propyl ester
PG
Progallin

Progallin P
Tenox PG
3,4,5,-Trihydroxybenzoic acid, propyl ester
Uantox PG

Uses

1. Foods
2. Medicines
3. Cosmetics (lipsticks and moisturizers)

Prevention

Propyl gallate is one of the family of gallate ester chemicals that includes octyl and dodecyl gallate. They are used in the food, pharmaceutical, and cosmetic industries as an antioxidant to prevent oils and fats from becoming rancid. It is unlikely that foods containing this substance are causing your dermatitis. By reading labels on cosmetics and medicines, avoidance of skin contact with these gallate compounds should be possible.

May be duplicated for use in clinical practice. From Marks JG Jr, Elsner P, DeLeo VA: *Contact and occupational dermatology,* ed 3, St Louis, 2002, Mosby.

Clinical Aspects

Propyl gallate is a member of the group of gallate esters that are used to prevent the oxidation of fatty acids into rancid smelling smaller compounds. The cosmetic, food, and pharmaceutical industries use these compounds frequently. Most cases of allergic contact dermatitis to the gallate esters have been to propyl gallate found in lipsticks, moisturizers, antibiotic creams, eye cosmetics, and body lotions. Despite its moderate sensitizing capability in guinea pigs, allergic contact dermatitis to propyl gallate has been reported only sporadically in humans. One report, however, suggests that the allergic potential of propyl gallate can be boosted by its attachment on liposomes that were found in several cosmetics marketed for smooth complexions.

> **Propyl gallate is an antioxidant found in cosmetics, medicaments, and foods.**

BIBLIOGRAPHY

Corazza M, Mantovani L, Roveggio C Virgili A: Allergic contact dermatitis from propyl gallate, *Contact Dermatitis* 31:203-204, 1994.

Giordano-Labadie F, Schwarze HP, Bazex J: Allergic contact dermatitis from octyl gallate in lipstick, *Contact Dermatitis* 42:51, 2000.

Hernández N, Assier-Bonnet H, Terki N et al: Allergic contact dermatitis from propyl gallate in desonide cream (Locapred), *Contact Dermatitis* 36:111, 1997.

Marston S: Propyl gallate on liposomes, *Contact Dermatitis* 27:74-76, 1992.

Romaguera C, Vilaplana J: Contact dermatitis from gallates, *Am J Contact Dermat* 4:231-234, 1993.

PROPYLENE GLYCOL

Definition

Propylene glycol is an aliphatic alcohol that is odorless, colorless, viscous, and tasteless. It has widespread use in cosmetics, pharmaceuticals, and industry because of its solvent and humectant qualities. Some topical medicaments contain greater than 50% propylene glycol. The Cosmetic Ingredient Review Expect Panel concluded propylene glycol is safe for use in cosmetic products at concentrations up to 50%. The United States Food and Drug Administration granted propylene glycol "generally recognized as safe" (GRAS) status as a food additive. The North American Contact Dermatitis Group uses 30% propylene glycol in water for patch testing, with 3.8% of their patients having allergic reactions to this chemical (Marks and others, 2000).

Clinical Aspects

Patch testing with propylene glycol can be difficult because differentiation of allergic from irritant reactions is hard. The literature reveals a marked amount of contradiction concerning irritant versus allergic reactions because patch test concentrations of propylene glycol vary in different studies from 10% to 100%. Some authors recommend low concentrations between 1% and 10% in order to avoid irritant reactions. The North American Contact Dermatitis Group currently uses a 30% solution for patch testing. It is recommended that a higher concentration of propylene glycol be used for patch testing when there is a strong suspicion of al-

---

EXPOSURE LIST ▶ **PROPYLENE GLYCOL**

Synonyms and Other Names
1,2-Dihydroxypropane
1,2-Propanediol
Methyl glycol

Uses
Propylene glycol is used widely in medicines, cosmetics, and industry because of its solvent, humectant, and preservative properties and has the following applications:
1. Cosmetics (lipsticks, moisturizers, and liquid makeup)
2. Pharmaceuticals (topical corticosteroids, ear preparations, sterile lubricant jelly, electrocardiogram gels, and injectables [intramuscular and intravenous])
3. Varnishes and synthetic resins
4. Antifreeze and deicing compounds
5. Foods (solvents for colors and flavors, emulsifier [e.g., salad dressings])
6. Household cleaning products

Prevention
Avoidance of propylene glycol in cosmetics and topical medications requires reading labels and the package inserts and on occasion, direct communication with the manufacturer. Glycerin is an excellent substitute for propylene glycol in many formulations. Extremely sensitive individuals may have a flare-up of dermatitis after oral ingestion of foods or the use of oral, intramuscular, or intravenous medications containing propylene glycol.

May be duplicated for use in clinical practice. From Marks JG Jr, Elsner P, DeLeo VA: *Contact and occupational dermatology,* ed 3, St Louis, 2002, Mosby.

lergy and a negative reaction to 10% propylene glycol. Another confounding factor is the increased number of positive patch test responses produced in the winter months when irritation from this compound is increased. It is important not to over-interpret propylene glycol patch test reactions, since exposure to this chemical is widespread. Inappropriate over-interpretation of patch test results could result in a propylene glycol "cripple." It can be concluded that propylene glycol is certainly a mild irritant, but in a small percentage of cases it is also an allergen. It also causes nonimmunologic contact urticaria and subjective or sensory irritation. Positive patch test responses should be confirmed by repeat patch testing as well as testing with the actual product. In a subset of propylene glycol–allergic individuals, oral challenge produces a generalized dermatitis and flare-ups of previous patch test sites and healed dermatitis (Catanzaro and Smith, 1991; Funk and Maibach, 1994; Jackson, 1995; Wahlberg, 1994).

> **Positive patch test responses to propylene glycol should be interpreted cautiously, since irritant reactions are common.**

BIBLIOGRAPHY

Angelini G, Meneghini CL: Contact allergy from propylene glycol, *Contact Dermatitis* 7:197-198, 1981.

Catanzaro JM, Smith JG: Propylene glycol dermatitis, *J Am Acad Dermatol* 24:90-95, 1991.

Fan W, Kinnunen T, Niinimäki A et al: Skin reactions to glycols used in dermatological and cosmetic vehicles, *Am J Contact Dermat* 2:181-183, 1991.

Fisher AA: Propylene glycol dermatitis, *Cutis* 21:166-178, 1978.

Fisher AA: The management of propylene glycol–sensitive patients, *Cutis* 25:24-44, 1980.

Frosch PG, Pekar U, Enzmann H: Contact allergy to propylene glycol: do we use the appropriate test concentration? *Dermatol Clin* 8:111-113, 1990.

Funk JO, Maibach HI: Propylene glycol dermatitis: reevaluation of an old problem, *Contact Dermatitis* 31:236-241, 1994.

Hannuksela M, Forstrom L: Reactions to peroral propylene glycol, *Contact Dermatitis* 4:41-45, 1978.

Jackson EM: Propylene glycol: irritant, sensitizer, or neither? *Cosmetic Dermatology* 8;43-45, 1995.

Marks JG, Belsito DV, DeLeo VA et al: North American Contact Dermatitis Group standard tray patch test results: 1996 to 1998, *Arch Dermatol* 136:272-273, 2000.

Trancik RJ, Maibach HI: Propylene glycol: irritation or sensitization? *Contact Dermatitis* 8:185-189, 1982.

Wahlberg JE: Propylene glycol: search for a proper and nonirritant patch test preparation, *Am J Contact Dermat* 5:156-159, 1994.

POLYETHYLENE GLYCOLS

Definition

Polyethylene glycols (PEGs) are clear, viscous liquids and white, solid polymers of ethylene oxide. They are used extensively in cosmetics and topical medicaments, and over 600 topical products contain PEGs. They are patch tested "as is" at 100% concentration. The North American Contact Dermatitis Group found 0.8% of their patients to be allergic to PEG 400 (Marks and others, 1995).

BOX 7-1

Cosmetic Dermatitis

1. Fragrances and preservatives are the most common causes of cosmetic allergic contact dermatitis.
2. Neither the patient nor the physician is frequently aware that a cosmetic was the cause of allergic contact dermatitis before patch testing.
3. Skin care and hair products are the most common causes of contact dermatitis from cosmetics.
4. Adult women are most frequently affected.
5. The face and periorbital skin are most frequently affected.
6. Five percent of patch test clinic patients have allergic contact dermatitis from a cosmetic.

Table 7-2

Contact Dermatitis Due to Cosmetic Products

Product	North America* (%)	Netherlands† (%)
Skin care products	28	56
Hair products	25	6
Facial makeup	10	1
Nail preparations	8	13
Fragrance	7	8
Eye makeup	4	3
Personal cleanliness preparations	6	2
Shaving preparation	4	3
Other cosmetics	13	8

*North American Contact Dermatitis Group (Adams and others, 1985) (713 patients).
†deGroot, Bruynzell, Bos, 1988 (199 patients).

than 1% of these being allergic contact dermatitis. Most of the information concerning adverse cutaneous reactions from cosmetics comes from (1) case reports in the dermatologic literature, which are the harbingers of potentially significant allergens in a cosmetic formulation; (2) consumer reports to industry and government; and (3) contact dermatitis clinics. These sources of information must certainly underestimate the frequency of adverse reactions, since probably the majority of individuals with minor reactions simply tolerate or stop using the suspected product. Valid data for the frequency of allergic contact dermatitis due to cosmetic ingredients await a general population epidemiologic study. Despite this, two patch test clinic investigations, one in North America and the other in the Netherlands, have identified products (Table 7-2) and ingredients (Table 7-3) that are the most common causes of allergic contact dermatitis from cosmetics.

Table 7-3	Ingredients Causing Contact Dermatitis	
Ingredient	North America* (%)	Netherlands† (%)
Fragrance	30	27
Preservative	28	32
p-Phenylenediamine	8	–
Lanolin	5	3
Glyceryl thioglycolate	5	–
Propylene glycol	5	–
Tosylamide/formaldehyde resin	4	10
Sunscreens and ultraviolet absorbers	4	2
Acrylates	1	–
Others	10	26

*North American Contact Dermatitis Group (Adams and others, 1985) (713 patients).
†deGroot, Bruynzell, Bos, 1988 (199 patients).

Cosmetic intolerance syndrome is not a single entity.

One group of particularly difficult patients has the "cosmetic intolerance syndrome," or "status cosmeticus." These patients complain bitterly of facial burning and discomfort with or without facial inflammation. These individuals are no longer able to tolerate the use of any cosmetics. This syndrome is not made up of a single entity but can have multiple exogenous and endogenous origins, including irritant and allergic contact dermatitis, photoallergic contact dermatitis, contact urticaria, seborrheic dermatitis, psoriasis, rosacea, atopic dermatitis, and significant psychological disorder. The diagnosis and management of these patients require a detailed history, skin examination, testing for contact dermatitis and urticaria, use of bland topicals, and if necessary, treatment of psychiatric disorder.

Adverse cutaneous reactions to cosmetics are varied, including subjective and objective irritation, allergic contact dermatitis, contact urticaria, dyspigmentation, nail dystrophy, hair breakage, and acne. The main cosmetics causing irritant contact dermatitis include soaps and detergents, deodorants and antiperspirants, eye shadow, mascara, shampoos, permanent hair-waving products, and moisturizers. The most common cosmetic allergens are fragrances, preservatives, and hair dyes (see Plates). Contact urticaria is caused by a number of cosmetic ingredients, including fragrances, preservatives, and particularly ammonium persulfate in hair bleaches. Contact urticaria is discussed further in Chapter 16. Hyperpigmentation of the face occurs more frequently in dark-complexioned individuals. Fragrances, perfumes, 0.1% or less; cosmetics, 0.5%; colognes, 4%; toilet water, 5%; and perfumes, 20%. Perfumery is both an art and a science, with the perfumer combining the biochemistry of fragrance ingredients with the artistry of blending aromas. A typical fragrance formula contains 10 to 300 individual ingredients; some perfumes can contain up to 800.

Hands, face, legs, and axillae are common sites affected by allergic contact dermatitis from fragrances.

The most common adverse cutaneous reaction to fragrances is allergic contact dermatitis (see Plates). Photodermatitis, contact urticaria, irritation, depigmentation, and hyperpigmentation are occasionally seen. The North American Contact Dermatitis Group study (Adams and others, 1985) of cosmetic reactions found that fragrances were the most common ingredient causing cutaneous reactions. Another important finding of this study was that half of the patients or physicians were unaware that a cosmetic was responsible for the dermatitis. Most of the fragrance reactions were from unspecified fragrances. Individual fragrance allergens identified in decreasing order of frequency were cinnamic alcohol, hydroxycitronellal, musk ambrette, isoeugenol, geraniol, cinnamic aldehyde, coumarin, and eugenol. Oak moss is the most common allergen, with marked reduction of sensitivity to cinnamic alcohol and cinnamic aldehyde. It is often difficult to investigate a suspected fragrance contact dermatitis, since there may be hundreds of fragrance ingredients and the availability of fragrance allergens is limited.

Fragrances are the most common cosmetic ingredient causing allergic contact dermatitis.

The perfume screening series that was distributed by the American Academy of Dermatology is no longer available in the United States. It contained six of the common fragrance allergens: cinnamic alcohol, cinnamic aldehyde, eugenol, hydroxycitronellal, isoeugenol, and oak moss absolute. Seven less common fragrance allergens on the tray were alphaamylcinnamic alcohol, anisyl alcohol, benzyl alcohol, benzyl salicylate, coumarin, geraniol, and sandalwood oil. One photoallergen, musk ambrette, was also included. Fragrance mixtures have also been used for screening patients suspected of having fragrance allergies. The perfume mixture was deleted from the American Academy of Dermatology standard tray because of frequent false-positive reactions due to irritant contact dermatitis. The International Contact Dermatitis Research Group reduced the patch test concentrations of the eight individual fragrances in the mixture from 2% to 1% to reduce false-positive reactions. Balsam of Peru and wood tars are also used as markers of fragrance sensitivity. Balsam of Peru and fragrance mix are standard-tray allergens and are discussed in Chapter 5. Musk ambrette, 6-methylcoumarin, and sandalwood oil are photoallergens and are reviewed in Chapter 9.

> **Balsam of Peru and fragrance mix are present in the standard tray. These mixtures identify approximately 50% and 75%, respectively, of the patients with fragrance sensitivity.**

Strategies have been implemented to reduce the sensitizing potential of fragrance materials. These include (1) eliminating or reducing the concentration of known sensitizers, (2) use of safe alternatives, (3) use of pure, standardized fragrance materials, and (4) formulation of products that contain ingredients that may inhibit sensitization ("quenching" agents). For example, cinnamic aldehyde, which is a strong sensitizer, when formulated with an equal weight of eugenol (quencher), prevents sensitization. The quenching phenomenon of delayed contact hypersensitivity, however, has been questioned by some investigators.

> **Since individual fragrances are not listed on the cosmetic label, a use test should be performed before starting to use a new perfumed product.**

The fragrance industry has established a system of self-regulation. The International Fragrance Association (IFRA) publishes a code of practice for the industry and guidelines for ingredient usage (Table 7-4). These guidelines rely on data provided by industry, academia, and the Research Institute of Fragrance Materials (RIFM), 375 Sylvan Avenue, Englewood Cliffs, NJ. The RIFM carries out research for the sole purpose of establishing data on the toxicologic effects of fragrance raw materials.

Table 7-4	International Fragrance Association (IFRA) Industry Guidelines to Restrict Ingredient Usage*
Selected Fragrances	**Comment**
Cinnamic alcohol	Should not be used as a fragrance ingredient at a level over 4% in fragrance compounds.
Cinnamic aldehyde	Use in conjunction with substances preventing sensitization (e.g., equal weights of eugenol and d-limonene).
Colophony	Should not be used as a fragrance ingredient.
Dihydrocoumarin	Should not be used as a fragrance ingredient.
7-Methylcoumarin	Should not be used as a fragrance ingredient.
Hydroxycitronellal	Should not be used as a fragrance ingredient at a level over 5% in fragrance compounds.
Isoeugenol	Should not be used as a fragrance ingredient at a level over 1% in fragrance compounds.
Musk ambrette	Should not be used as a fragrance ingredient.
Balsam of Peru	Should not be used as a fragrance ingredient.
Oak moss absolute	Should not be used in fragrance compounds at levels over 3%.

*Extracted from the International Fragrance Association (IFRA) Code of Practice.

> **Fragrances are the most frequent cause of allergic contact dermatitis from cosmetics, and cinnamic aldehyde is one of the most common fragrance allergens.**

Clinical Aspects

Cinnamic aldehyde is an aromatic chemical found in cinnamon leaves, cinnamon bark, and the essential oils of hyacinth, myrrh, Bulgarian rose, patchouli, and other plants. The amount of cinnamic aldehyde varies considerably among the botanic species. For example, Chinese cinnamon bark oil (oil of cassia) has 70% to 90% cinnamic aldehyde, whereas Ceylon cinnamon leaf oil has less than 7%.

EXPOSURE LIST ▸ **CINNAMIC ALDEHYDE**

Synonyms and Other Names

Cinnamal
Cinnamaldehyde
3-Phenyl-2-propenal

Phenylacrolein
2-Propenal-3-phenyl

Uses

Cinnamic aldehyde has a sweet, spicy odor typical of cinnamon. It is a perfume and flavor chemical used in the following products:

1. Perfumes and fragrances
2. Toothpaste and mouthwash
3. Balsam of Tolu and balsam of Peru
4. Plants such as hyacinth
5. Cinnamon, Ceylon, and cassia oil
6. Fragranced household products such as deodorizers, detergents, and soaps
7. Foods: Cola, chocolate, ice cream, chewing gums, candy
8. Spices
9. Cosmetics
10. Medicated creams and ointments

Prevention

Allergic contact dermatitis from cinnamic aldehyde principally occurs from fragrances in cosmetics and household products. It is also a flavoring, particularly in toothpaste. Because perfumes and fragrances contain dozens of chemicals, a listing of the individual ingredients, such as cinnamic aldehyde, is not given. Thus an individual must avoid all fragranced cosmetics to be certain to prevent allergic contact dermatitis that is due to cinnamic aldehyde. Because of the quenching phenomenon, however, perfumes that do contain cinnamic aldehyde may be tolerated by individuals who are sensitive to this chemical. Pretesting with the fragrance prior to use is important and is done by applying a small amount on a limited area of the forearm twice daily for 1 week. Another ploy is to use perfume on hair or clothing rather than in direct skin contact. Toothpastes that do not contain cinnamic aldehyde include regular Colgate.

Bakers may develop hand dermatitis due to this chemical from spices used in cooking. A generalized dermatitis from ingestion of foods and spices containing cinnamic aldehyde is quite uncommon.

May be duplicated for use in clinical practice. From Marks JG Jr, Elsner P, DeLeo VA: *Contact and occupational dermatology,* ed 3, St Louis, 2002, Mosby.

Cinnamic aldehyde is used as a fragrance in cosmetics and over-the-counter drugs and as a flavoring agent in beverages, chewing gum, mouthwashes, and toothpaste. Synthetic cinnamic aldehyde (cinnamaldehyde) is manufactured by the condensation of acetaldehyde with benzaldehyde. Its concentration varies from 0.03% in creams to 0.1% in perfumes.

Cinnamic aldehyde is an irritant and strong sensitizer and has caused contact urticaria. When patch tested at an 8% concentration in petrolatum, it is a strong irritant. Both animal and human studies have shown it to be a strong sensitizer. There is cross-reactivity among cinnamic aldehyde, cinnamic alcohol, and cinnamic acid, with cinnamic aldehyde being the strongest sensitizer. It is believed that cinnamic aldehyde is the true allergen among these chemicals. Cinnamic alcohol and cinnamic acid are "prohaptens" that are transformed within the skin to cinnamic aldehyde before causing allergic contact dermatitis. It is also now thought that the binding sites of cinnamic aldehyde on the protein carrier are with the thiol groups of cysteine residues rather than the amino groups of lysine residues.

Schorr (1975) found positive patch test responses to this fragrance in 2.8% of 34 males and 9.1% of 55 females that may have been traceable to perfumed cosmetics. In a Danish manufacturing firm almost all workers who were exposed to high concentrations of cinnamon spice substitute developed allergies to cinnamic aldehyde. Oral symptoms from toothpaste containing cinnamic aldehyde include sore mouth, dermatitis of the lips and perioral skin, swelling of the tongue, and mouth ulceration.

The "quenching" phenomenon is a consistent finding whereby cinnamic aldehyde alone induces sensitization but when mixed with other fragrance compounds such as eugenol or d-limonene induces no sensitization. Patients who are sensitive to cinnamic aldehyde can sometimes tolerate perfumes containing this allergen because of presumed chemical changes (quenching) that occur during the usual aging process of a "mature" perfume. The International Fragrance Association recommends that cinnamic aldehyde be used with an equal proportion by weight of eugenol or d-limonene to prevent sensitization.

BIBLIOGRAPHY

Collins FW, Mitchell JC: Aroma chemicals, *Contact Dermatitis* 1:43-47, 1975.

Fisher AA, Dooms-Goossens A: The effect of perfume "ageing" on the allergenicity of individual perfume ingredients, *Contact Dermatitis* 2:155-159, 1976.

Guin JD: Cinnamic aldehyde. In Guin JB, editor: *Practical contact dermatitis: a handbook for the practitioner,* New York, 1995, McGraw-Hill.

Magnusson B, Wilkinson DS: Cinnamic aldehyde in toothpaste, *Contact Dermatitis* 1:70-80, 1975.

Majeti VA, Suskind RR: Mechanism of cinnamaldehyde sensitization, *Contact Dermatitis* 3:16-18, 1977.

Opdyke DLJ: Cinnamic aldehyde, *J Food Cosmetics Toxicol* 17:253-258, 1979.

Sainio EL, Kanerva L: Contact allergens in toothpastes and a review of their hypersensitivity, *Contact Dermatitis* 33:100-105, 1995.

Schorr WF: Cinnamic aldehyde allergy, *Contact Dermatitis* 1:108-111, 1975.

Weibel H, Hansen J: Interaction of cinnamaldehyde (a sensitizer in fragrance) with protein, *Contact Dermatitis* 20:161-166, 1989.

Weibel H, Hansen J, Andersen KE: Cross-sensitization patterns in guinea pigs between cinnamaldehyde, cinnamyl alcohol and cinnamic acid, *Acta Derm Venereol Suppl (Stockh)* 69:302-307, 1989.

Hair Care Product Allergens ▬▬▬

Hair care products are frequent causes of contact dermatitis in clients and beauticians (Plates 12, 21, and 24). In the North American Contact Dermatitis Group cosmetic study (Adams and others, 1985), 25% of the reactions were caused by hair care products that included shampoos, rinses, hair sprays, permanent hair-waving preparations, hair dyes, and bleaches. Shampoos are a frequent cause of irritant contact dermatitis in hairdressers because the shampoos remove protective skin lipids and have a drying action on the hands. *p*-Phenylenediamine, the allergen in permanent hair dyes, is the third most common ingredient after fragrances and preservatives to cause allergic contact dermatitis from cosmetics. *p*-Phenylenediamine is discussed in Chapter 5, since it is a standard allergen. The other significant allergen in hair care products, *glyceryl thioglycolate,* which is found in permanent hair-waving preparations, is discussed below. *Ammonium persulfate* is added to hair bleaches as an oxidizer to boost and accelerate the bleaching process. It has been reported to cause contact urticaria, generalized urticarial reactions, and asthma.

> **Ammonium persulfate, used to "boost" peroxide hair bleaches, causes contact urticaria and anaphylactoid reactions.**

GLYCERYL THIOGLYCOLATE

Definition

Glyceryl thioglycolate (glyceryl monothioglycolate) is the monoester of glycerin and thioglycolic acid and is used in acid permanents to alter the curvature of the hair. It is a more frequent sensitizer of cosmetologists than of patrons who have hair permanents. It was the fifth most common cause of dermatitis in the 5-year North American Contact Dermatitis study of cosmetic reactions (Adams and others, 1985). A 1% concentration of glyceryl thioglycolate in petrolatum is recommended for patch testing. The North American Contact Dermatitis Group found 1.9% of their patch test clinic patients allergic to this chemical (Marks and others, 2000).

> **Glyceryl thioglycolate (monothioglycolate), the allergen in acid permanents, causes allergic contact dermatitis in hairdressers and their clients.**

Clinical Aspects

Permanent hair-waving solutions alter the curvature of the hair by breaking disulfide bonds within the keratin structure of the hair shaft. This allows softening and assumption of the new shape, which is held permanently by rebonding of the disulfide bonds. Two types of permanent hair-waving chemicals are used to accomplish this. The older, *alkaline permanents* containing *ammonium thioglycolate* are used at home and by salon hairdressers. Ammonium thioglycolate is a known irritating chemical that, if allowed to have prolonged or repeated skin con-

---

EXPOSURE LIST ▶ **GLYCEROL THIOGLYCOLATE**

Synonyms and Other Names

Acetic acid, mercapto-, monoester with
  1,2,3-propanetriol
Acid permanent waves
Glycerol monomercaptoacetate

Glyceryl monothioglycolate
Hot permanent waves
Mercaptoacetic acid, monoester with 1,2,3-propanetriol

Uses

Glyceryl thioglycolate is the essential ingredient in acid permanent hair-waving solutions.

Prevention

Glyceryl thioglycolate can be avoided by not using permanent hair-waving solutions that contain this chemical. These solutions are found only in salons in the United States and are usually referred to as acid or hot permanents. These permanents can be identified because the packages usually contain three bottles or containers. There is no cross-reactivity with ammonium thioglycolate, the active ingredient in alkaline permanents, which can be recognized because these preparations contain only two bottles or containers. Salon product labeling, which is voluntarily being introduced in the United States, should help hairdressers and clients to avoid glyceryl thioglycolate. Hair that has been permed with glyceryl thioglycolate may have persistence of the allergen for at least 3 months after the permanent, and this can cause long-lasting dermatitis in clients or beauticians. Glyceryl thioglycolate easily penetrates through many rubber and vinyl gloves, which makes it difficult to impossible for beauticians to continue permanent hair-waving with this allergen.

May be duplicated for use in clinical practice. From Marks JG Jr, Elsner P, DeLeo VA: *Contact and occupational dermatology,* ed 3, St Louis, 2002, Mosby.

---

tact, causes irritant contact dermatitis in clients or hairdressers, or both. Because it is irritating, ammonium thioglycolate is difficult to patch test, and reports of allergic contact dermatitis from this chemical have been questioned.

More recently, *acid permanents* containing *glyceryl thioglycolate* were introduced only as a salon product to be used by cosmetologists. Several reports have confirmed that it is a significant allergen for hairdressers and also for clients. Storrs (1984) reported eight hairdressers and four clients who were allergic to the glyceryl thioglycolate found in acid permanents that they had used. Because of unexplained persistence of dermatitis in beauty shop clients or recurrent allergic contact dermatitis in hairdressers, further investigation showed that either glyceryl thioglycolate or its by-products remain in the hair shaft for months after the permanent. Controversy concerning the allergic nature of glyceryl thioglycolate exists, since it is unstable and can readily break down to form the irritant thioglycolic acid. The North American Contact Dermatitis Group and others, however, have found that glyceryl thioglycolate, 1% in petrolatum, is not an irritant and gives many relevant positive patch test reactions (Marks and others, 1995).

Glyceryl thioglycolate or its by-products can remain in the hair shaft for months, causing chronic allergic contact dermatitis.

Allergic contact dermatitis resulting from topical corticosteroids was until recently thought to be a relatively rare phenomenon. In some countries frequency of allergic contact dermatitis to these agents is now similar to that for standard allergens. It usually develops in the setting of chronic dermatitis, like stasis eczema or atopic dermatitis. The patient usually notes a failure to clear or a flare-up of the eczema being treated with a topical corticosteroid. In addition, facial dermatitis from corticosteroid allergy to nasal spray is becoming more common. Diagnosing allergic contact dermatitis requires a high level of suspicion by the clinician, which leads to patch testing. In the vast majority of cases the etiologic agent in the topical corticosteroid is a preservative or vehicle component rather than the corticosteroid itself; in fact, patients who are allergic to corticosteroids frequently are also allergic to components of topical medicaments.

Patch testing to corticosteroids is complicated by the therapeutic, antiinflammatory nature of the corticosteroid itself, which results in frequent false-negative findings. The corticosteroid may inhibit the allergic response itself in the patch test procedure. Unlike many antigens that produce false-positive or irritant responses when tested at too high a concentration, corticosteroids may inhibit the response and result in a false-negative response when tested at too high a concentration. Therefore it is essential that agents be tested at the proper concentration. The vehicle of the patch test may also play a role in the ability to obtain a positive response in allergic individuals. Ethanol seems to be preferable, but many corticosteroids are not stable in ethanol, so petrolatum is frequently used. For testing to marketed agents it is better to test in a cream base rather than in an ointment base. As yet, there are no standard concentrations and vehicles that are known to be optimal. However, most authorities agree that testing with tixocortal pivilate, budesonide, and hydrocortison-17-butyrate would represent a good screening panel.

True allergy to corticosteroids may be evidenced by a "reverse edge effect" on patch testing, which occurs when the therapeutic activity of the agent causes a negative response directly under the disk of the test with a positive eczematous response at the edge or surrounding the disk application site. Positive reactions to corticosteroids may also be markedly delayed (5 to 7 days before a positive reading).

Extensive cross-reactivity among different corticosteroids is reported. An investigation of this phenomenon and related structural differences has led to grouping of agents into the four classes listed in Table 8-1. Agents within a group would be expected to cross-react. Cross-reactivity among groups is less likely but may occur, especially to classes B and D. An individual found to be sensitive to one agent in a group should be instructed to avoid the other agents in that group. Testing such a patient to selected corticosteroids from the other groups helps define what agents can be used safely by an allergic individual. It should be noted that reactions have occurred to systemic and intraarticular usage of agents to which a patient was sensitized topically. Therefore patients must be instructed to avoid corticosteroid administration by routes other than the topical one.

Most corticosteroids are available in the United States by prescription only. Two agents, hydrocortisone and hydrocortisone acetate, are available without prescription.

EXPOSURE LIST ▷ CORTICOSTEROIDS

Synonyms and Other Names

Class A: Hydrocortisone and tixocortol type
  Cortisone
  Cortisone acetate
  Hydrocortisone
  Hydrocortisone acetate
  Methylprednisolone
  Methylprednisone acetate
  Prednisolone
  Prednisolone acetate
  Tixocortol pivalate
Class B: Triamcinolone acetonide type
  Triamcinolone acetonide
  Triamcinolone alcohol
  Halcinonide
  Flucinonide
  Fluocinolone acetonide
  Desonide
  Budesonide
  Amcinonide

Class C: Betamethasone type
  Betamethasone
  Betamethasone–disodium phosphate
  Dexamethasone
  Dexamethasone–disodium phosphate
  Fluocortolone
Class D: Hydrocortisone-17-butyrate and clobetasone-17-butyrate type
  Hydrocortisone butyrate
  Hydrocortisone valerate
  Clobetasone butyrate
  Clobetasol propionate
  Betamethasone valerate
  Betamethasone dipropionate
  Fluocortolone hexanoate
  Fluocortolone pivalate
  Prednicarbate
  Alclometasone dipropionate

Uses

Corticosteroid agents are used extensively in medicine and dentistry. They can be administered by infusion and injection, by mouth, by respiratory and nasal inhaler, by enema, in eye and ear drops and ointments, and in creams, lotions, ointments, and tapes for skin application. Most of these are prescription products in the United States (except class A).

Prevention

Patients allergic to some corticosteroids should be told which of these four previously described classes of agents they should avoid. Because almost all of these are available only by prescription, allergic individuals should be instructed to inform all their health care providers of their allergies and give them a copy of this sheet for the medical records.

Because two products in class A are available without a prescription—hydrocortisone and hydrocortisone acetate—the ingredient list of any medicated cream, lotion, or the like should be examined before purchasing, to be certain that it does not contain either agent.

Individuals who are allergic to agents in class B may also react to agents in class D.

May be duplicated for use in clinical practice. From Marks JG Jr, Elsner P, DeLeo VA: *Contact and occupational dermatology,* ed 3, St Louis, 2002, Mosby.

BIBLIOGRAPHY

Coopman S, Degreef H, Dooms-Goossens A: Identification of cross-reaction patterns in allergic contact dermatitis from topical corticosteroids, *Br J Dermatol* 121:27-34, 1989.

Cronin E: *Contact dermatitis,* London, 1980, Churchill Livingstone.

Dooms-Goosens A: Contact dermatitis to topical corticosteroids: diagnostic problems. In *Exogenous dermatoses: environmental dermatitis,* Boca Raton, Fla, 1991, CRC Press.

Dooms-Goossens A: Corticosteroid contact allergy: a challenge to patch testing, *Am J Contact Dermat* 4:120-122, 1993.

Dooms-Goossens A, Degreef H, Parijs M et al: A retrospective study of patch test results from 163 patients with stasis dermatitis or leg ulcers, *Dermatologica* 159:93-106, 1979.

Feldman SB, Sexton FM, Busas J et al: Allergic contact dermatitis from topical steroids, *Contact Dermatitis* 19:226-228, 1988.

Fortstrom L, Lassus A, Salde L et al: Allergic contact eczema from topical corticosteroids, *Contact Dermatitis* 8:128-133, 1982.

Guin Jere D: Contact sensitivity to topical steroids, *J Am Acad Dermatol* 5:773-782, 1984.

Rietschel RL, Fowler JF: *Fisher's contact dermatitis,* ed 4, Philadelphia, 1995, Lea & Febiger.

GENTAMICIN SULFATE

Definition

Gentamicin sulfate (Garamycin) is an antibiotic used topically and parenterally, but not orally. It is tested at 20% concentration in petrolatum. Although no prevalence studies have been reported, it is thought to be a rare primary sensitizer. Cross-reactivity between gentamicin and neomycin is common.

Clinical Aspects

Gentamicin is an antibiotic complex produced by *Micromonospora purpurea* or *Micromonospora echinospora.* It is a broad-spectrum antibiotic that is ineffective via the oral route but is used parenterally and in skin and ophthalmologic preparations. Such topical preparations are single-agent ones containing gentamicin at 0.1% concentration and are available only by prescription in the United States.

Parenteral use of gentamicin may result in deafness and renal damage. There is a report of tinnitus associated with topical usage.

EXPOSURE LIST ▷ **GENTAMICIN SULFATE**

Synonyms and Other Names

Cidomycin   Gentalyn
Garamycin   Refobacin
Gentacin

Uses

Gentamicin sulfate is used as an antibiotic for intravenous and topical use. It is available only by prescription in the United States and has the following applications:
1. Intravenous antibiotics
2. Cream and ointment medications
3. Eyedrops and ointments

Prevention

Patients who are allergic to gentamicin should be instructed to make all their health care providers aware of the allergy. They may also be allergic to neomycin and kanamycin, so they should read the labels of all medications made for the skin, eyes, and ears and avoid those that contain neomycin, kanamycin, or gentamicin and the substances named above.

> **Gentamicin sulfate (Garamycin) is a rare primary sensitizer. However, many patients who are allergic to neomycin sulfate, a common sensitizer, also react to gentamicin.**

Gentamicin is thought to be a rare primary sensitizer. Most cases of positive patch test responses to this agent are reported to be due to cross-reactivity with neomycin as the primary sensitizer. In one study, 40 of 100 patients who were sensitized to neomycin were found to be patch test–positive to gentamicin, even though the patients had no previous exposure to gentamicin.

Primary gentamicin sensitivity has been reported in patients with stasis dermatitis who received treatment with the agent and through occupational contact in a hospital laboratory worker.

BIBLIOGRAPHY

Cronin E: *Contact dermatitis,* London, 1980, Churchill Livingstone.

Drake TE: Reaction to gentamicin sulfate cream, *Arch Dermatol* 110:638-642, 1974.

Prila V, Hirvonen ML, Rouhunkoski S: The pattern of cross-sensitivity to neomycin: secondary sensitization to gentamicin, *Dermatologica* 136:321-326, 1968.

Rietschel RL, Fowler JF: *Fisher's contact dermatitis,* ed 4, Philadelphia, 1995, Lea & Febiger.

NITROFURAZONE (FURACIN)

Definition

Nitrofurazone (Furacin) is a topical antimicrobial agent that is used primarily to treat skin disease, burns, and injuries and is a potent sensitizer. It is tested at a concentration of 1% in petrolatum.

Clinical Aspects

Nitrofurazone is an antimicrobial agent used topically and is available as a powder, a cream, and an impregnated dressing. Because of its broad-spectrum antibacterial activity, Furacin is frequently used to treat severe burns, skin wounds, and ulcers in the hospital setting. The cream preparation of nitrofurazone has been used extensively in Europe to treat stasis dermatitis.

Nitrofurazone is a potent sensitizer. The overall incidence of contact allergy is estimated to be 1% of those who use a Furacin preparation. In addition to the high incidence of sensitization, the reported reactions are noted to be particularly severe and require hospitalization and systemic corticosteroid therapy in some cases.

The Furacin preparations contain polyethylene glycols, which may also cause allergic contact dermatitis. Nitrofurazone is also used in veterinary medicine and in animal feed.

> **Nitrofurazone (Furacin) is a potent sensitizer. The allergic contact dermatitis produced by this agent may be severe.**

EXPOSURE LIST ▸ **NITROFURAZONE (Furacin)**

Synonyms and Other Names

Aldomycin

Amifur

Chemofuran

Coxistat

Furacin

Mammex

Nifuzon

Nitrofural

5-Nitro-2-furaldehyde semicarbazone

Vabrocid

Uses

Nitrofurazone is used as a topical antibiotic and has the following applications:

1. Ointment and cream medications
2. Powder medications
3. Medicated dressings
4. Animal feed

Prevention

Patients allergic to nitrofurazone should be instructed to make their health care providers aware of their allergy. Labels of all skin medications should be examined to avoid those that contain nitrofurazone and substances named above. Animal feeds and veterinary medications may also contain nitrofurazone.

May be duplicated for use in clinical practice. From Marks JG Jr, Elsner P, DeLeo VA: *Contact and occupational dermatology,* ed 3, St Louis, 2002, Mosby.

BIBLIOGRAPHY

Cronin E: *Contact dermatitis,* London, 1980, Churchill Livingstone.

Hall PR, Beer HAD: Topical nitrofurazone: a potent sensitizer of the skin and mucosa, *S Afr Med J* 52:189-196, 1977.

Rietschel RL, Fowler JF: *Fisher's contact dermatitis,* ed 4, Philadelphia, 1995, Lea & Febiger.

PROPOLIS

Definition

Propolis, or *bee glue,* is a resin obtained from beehives. It is widely used as a component of homeopathic medications for both oral and topical administration. An uncommon sensitizer, it is tested at 10% concentration in petrolatum.

Clinical Aspects

Propolis is a resinous substance that is collected from tree buds by bees. The bees use the material in building hives by combining it with beeswax to make a cementing substance. Extraction of the natural product yields propolis wax, propolis resin, and propolis balsam. Propolis contains cinnamic acid and alcohol, as well as vanillin.

Propolis is the most common cause of occupational contact allergy in beekeepers. It is a much more common sensitizer than beeswax. Used extensively as a homeopathic medicament, propolis is sold (primarily in health food stores) as a "pure" solid in chunks and tablets to be chewed. It is also combined with other ingredients to make topical agents, including creams, ointments, and powders both for cosmetic and purported therapeutic usage, and it has been used as an anesthetic. Propolis has been used as a leather and wood varnish.

<table>
<tr><td>EXPOSURE LIST ▶ PROPOLIS</td></tr>
</table>

Synonyms and Other Names

Bee bread	Propolis balsam
Bee glue	Propolis resin
Hive doss	Propolis wax

Uses

Propolis is used as a homeopathic medication and is derived from beehives. It has the following applications:

1. Tablets
2. Chunks for chewing
3. Ointments
4. Powders
5. Varnish
6. Beehives

Prevention

Patients who are allergic to propolis should be instructed to read the labels of the previously listed agents and avoid those that contain propolis or synonymous substances. If patients also react adversely to fragrances, they must avoid all fragrance-containing products. Allergic beekeepers will have to avoid contact with beehives or use rubber gloves for all such contact.

––––––––

May be duplicated for use in clinical practice. From Marks JG Jr, Elsner P, DeLeo VA: *Contact and occupational dermatology,* ed 3, St Louis, 2002, Mosby.

Chewing propolis has led to the development of stomatitis and perioral dermatitis.

Because of its derivation from plant resins, propolis contains and/or cross-reacts with balsam of Peru and many other fragrances, including cinnamates and eugenol. The antigen has been identified as the dimethylallyl ester of caffeic acid.

BIBLIOGRAPHY

Cronin E: *Contact dermatitis,* London, 1980, Churchill Livingstone.

Hausen BM, Wollenweber E, Senff H et al: Propolis allergy, *Contact Dermatitis* 17:163-170, 1987.

Rietschel RL, Fowler JF: *Fisher's contact dermatitis,* ed 4, Philadelphia, 1995, Lea & Febiger.

RESORCINOL

Definition

Resorcinol (Resorcin) is a keratolytic that is used primarily in the treatment of acne and as a component of Castellani's paint for the treatment of intertriginous fungal infection. A rare sensitizer, it is tested at 2% concentration in petrolatum.

Clinical Aspects

Resorcinol is a benzenediol, *m*-dihydroxybenzene. It was once a common component of topical products used to treat acne. This usage was based on its keratolytic properties. The use of resorcinol has declined with the advent of topical antibiotics and benzoyl peroxides as therapeutic agents for the treatment of acne.

The other major source of exposure to resorcinol is in the medicament Castellani's paint, a long-standing treatment for macerated, mixed fungal, yeast, and bacterial infections in web spaces and intertriginous areas. Usage of this agent has also declined significantly in the last two decades.

Resorcinol is also present in a number of cosmetics, including skin fresheners, hair dyes and tonics, eye drops, and freckle creams. It is combined with benzocaine in antiitch preparations. It is present in some antihemorrhoidal suppositories.

Resorcinol is a component of a number of industrial processes, including the production of dyes, plastics, rubber, explosives, and celluloid. It is used in tanning leather, photocopying and photographic development, duplicating fluid, and mildew-proofing agents.

EXPOSURE LIST ▶ RESORCINOL

Synonyms and Other Names
Resorcin
1,3-Benzenediol
m-Dihydroxybenzene

Uses
Resorcinol is used in topical medicaments, industrial processes, and personal care products, such as the following:
1. Acne treatments
2. Castellani's paint
3. Cosmetics
4. Hair dyes and tonics
5. Eye drops
6. Suppositories
Less common uses include the following:
1. Photocopying, photographic, and duplicating solutions
2. Plastic
3. Rubber
4. Leather
5. Explosives
6. Celluloid
7. Dyes

Prevention
Because resorcinol is used in medications, patients who are allergic to resorcinol should be instructed to inform their health care providers of their allergy. The labels of all medications and the cosmetics listed earlier should be read carefully to avoid resorcinol-containing products. Persons involved in the workplace with the production of any of the previously listed products may be exposed to resorcinol. In addition, allergic individuals should be instructed to avoid products for skin application or oral medications that contain hexylresorcinol and resorcinol monoacetate.

May be duplicated for use in clinical practice. From Marks JG Jr, Elsner P, DeLeo VA: *Contact and occupational dermatology,* ed 3, St Louis, 2002, Mosby.

Resorcinol may cross-react with hexylresorcinol, resorcinol monoacetate (Euresol), and 5-methylresorcinol (orcinol) and less frequently with phenol, hydroxyquinone, pyrocatechol, and pyrogallol. Resorcinol monoacetate is used in skin and scalp lotions. Hexaresorcinol is used in oral preparations—including sore-throat lozenges and troches, mouthwashes, and gargles, and as an anthelmintic. Such systemic usage can induce systemic contact dermatitis in sensitive individuals.

The most common source of sensitivity to resorcinol is Castellani's paint, which is also used as a skin marker in radiation oncology.

BIBLIOGRAPHY

Cronin E: *Contact dermatitis,* London, 1980, Churchill Livingstone.

Fisher AA: Resorcinol: a rare sensitizer, *Cutis* 29:331, 1982.

Rietschel RL, Fowler JF: *Fisher's contact dermatitis,* ed 4, Philadelphia, 1995, Lea & Febiger.

TRANSDERMAL DRUG DELIVERY SYSTEMS

Over the last 10 years a number of drugs traditionally administered by systemic routes have been packaged in transdermal delivery systems. Such systems allow for systemic absorption through the skin and achieve serum levels comparable to those for systemic administration. The advantages of transdermal delivery include elimination of local gastrointestinal tract irritation, continuous and sustained serum drug levels, and avoidance of hepatic "first-pass" metabolism. The most frequent disadvantages of such delivery are dermatologic, primarily irritant and allergic contact dermatitis.

Scopolamine, clonidine, estradiol, nitroglycerin, fentanyl, testosterone, nicotine, and isosorbide dinitrate are presently marketed in transdermal systems. When allergic contact dermatitis due to the device occurs, the sensitizer may be the drug itself or some component of the delivery system, including the adhesives, the reservoir, or the backing material.

Contact allergy to the active drug has been reported with scopolamine, clonidine, and nitroglycerin. Allergy to the estradiol system was usually attributable to components of the device and only rarely to the active drug.

Scopolamine produced sensitization in 10% of a group of sailors using the drug for prolonged periods. Clonidine was even more sensitizing; it induced contact allergy in up to 50% of patients using the system.

Patients who are sensitized topically to scopolamine and nitroglycerin can apparently take these drugs orally without developing dermatitis. Rarely have individuals with clonidine sensitization developed dermatitis on oral challenge.

Suggested patch test concentrations for active agents are as follows:

Clonidine, 9% in petrolatum or aqueous

Nitroglycerin, 0.2 mg/ml water

Scopolamine, 1% in water or petrolatum

Nicotine, 10% aqueous

Allergens within the delivery system include hydroxypropyl cellulose, methacrylates and ethanol.

BIBLIOGRAPHY

Hogan DJ, Maibach HI: Transdermal drug delivery systems: adverse reactions—dermatologic overview. In Menne T, Maibach HI, editors: *Exogenous dermatoses: environmental dermatitis,* Boca Raton, Fla, 1991, CRC Press.

Jordan W: Allergy and topical irritation associated with transdermal testosterone administration: a comparison of scrotal and nonscrotal transdermal systems, *Am J Contact Dermat* 8:108-113, 1997.

CHAPTER 9

Photoallergens

217

Table 9-1 — **Types of Exogenous Photochemical Sensitivity**

	Pathophysiology	
Route of Exposure	Toxic	Allergic
Topical	Photoirritant contact dermatitis	Photoallergic contact dermatitis
Systemic*	Phototoxicity to a systemic agent	Photoallergy to a systemic agent

*Photosensitivity to a systemic agent or a photodrug reaction.

Exogenous photochemical sensitivity is a term that is used to describe skin disease caused by the interaction of electromagnetic radiation and an exogenously acquired chemical agent. In all exogenous chemical photosensitivity responses both the chemical and radiation are necessary for the response to be produced. The exposure route can be either systemic or topical, and the mechanism of the response can be either irritant (toxic) or allergic (Table 9-1). This sensitivity results in four possible entities: photoirritant contact dermatitis (PICD), photoallergic contact dermatitis (PACD), photoallergy to a systemic agent, and phototoxicity to a systemic agent.

> **Photochemical sensitivity can be divided into photoallergic contact dermatitis, photoirritant contact dermatitis, and photosensitivity to a systemic agent.**

The distinction between the mechanism of action (allergic versus toxic) is a fairly easy one to make on the basis of clinical features in the case of topically applied chemicals. By definition, photo–patch testing to a chemical inducing PACD reveals positive responses only in sensitized individuals and negative responses in unsensitized individuals or the population in general. By contrast, all (or at least the vast majority) of the population develop positive reactions to photo–patch testing to a phototoxic agent (PICD). Other differences are outlined in Table 9-2. They include a reaction occurring on first exposure to the chemical agent and light in PICD, with a sensitization delay being necessary for PACD. The timing of the response to testing is delayed in PACD, as it is in allergic contact dermatitis. In PICD the timing of the response varies depending on the chemical involved; for instance, tars induce an immediate positive reaction in skin on exposure to radiation, whereas psoralens produce a response in skin 48 to 72 hours after exposure to light. On clinical and histologic examination PACD is evident as an eczematous response, whereas PICD results in erythema, edema, and bullous lesions on clinical examination and necrosis of keratinocytes on histologic study. The dose of both chemical and radiation necessary to induce the response is more critical to the production of PICD as compared with PACD.

The differences between phototoxicity and photoallergy to systemic agents are less clear, and such distinctions are usually based on animal and in vitro stud-

Table 9-2	Differences Between Photoallergic and Phototoxic Chemical Reactions	
Feature	**Photoallergic**	**Phototoxic**
Incidence	Low	High
Occurrence on first exposure	No	Yes
Onset after ultraviolet exposure	24-28 hours	Minutes to days
Dose dependence		
Chemical	Not crucial	Important
Radiation	Not crucial	Important
Clinical morphologic appearance	Eczematous (erythroderma)	Erythema and edema, bullous, eczematous, urticarial, papular, pigmentation, lichenoid, pseudoporphyric
Route of exposure		
Topical	+++	++
Systemic	+	+++

ies, not on a clinical basis. When the distinction has been made, almost all photosensitivity to systemic agents has been thought to be toxic in mechanism. In addition, most offending chemicals are therapeutic agents (Table 9-3). For these reasons it is convenient to refer to all such reactions as photosensitivity to a systemic agent (PSA) or as photodrug reactions.

Photoallergic contact dermatitis is diagnosed by photo–patch testing. Photoirritant contact dermatitis is diagnosed by history and clinical morphology (i.e., appearance).

The diagnosis of a photodrug reaction is made primarily by a history of ingestion of a photosensitizing agent and the presentation of a skin reaction in a photodistribution. Exposure of uninvolved skin to etiologic radiation while the patient is taking the drug may reproduce the eruption. Similarly, PICD is a diagnosis made by taking a careful history to reveal skin exposure to the photoirritant. Photo–patch testing in such patients is contraindicated because a positive response might be severe, would be expected to occur in the general population, and thus would not be helpful in making the diagnosis (Table 9-4).

The pathophysiologic mechanisms involved in PACD have been studied extensively. These studies routinely revealed that the immunologic process involved in this reaction is analogous to the process that occurs in plain allergic contact dermatitis to a nonphotosensitized antigen. The mechanism involved in the production of the photoantigen is less clearly defined.

Table 9-3	Common Drugs Inducing Photosensitivity to a Systemic Agent or Photodrug Reaction	
Antibiotics	Quinidine	
Griseofulvin	Diuretics	
Nalidixic acid	Furosemide	
Sulfanilamide	Hydrochlorothiazide	
Tetracyclines	Hematoporphyrin	
Ciprofloxacin	Nonsteroidal antiinflammatory drugs	
Chemotherapeutic agents	Benoxaprofen	
Dacarbazine	Piroxicam	
5-Fluorouracil	Naproxen	
Vinblastine	Psoralen	
Chlorpromazine	Tolbutamide	
Amiodarone		

Table 9-4	Agents Commonly Inducing Photoirritant Contact Dermatitis	
Tars	Plant products†	
Therapeutics	Lime	
Pitch, creosote	Celery	
Furocoumarins	Parsnip	
Therapeutics	Fig	
Fragrance materials*	Dyes	
	Eosin, methylene blue	
	Disperse blue 35	

*Berloque dermatitis.
†Phytophotodermatitis (not all-inclusive).

Ten to 20% of patients referred for phototesting because of a history of photosensitivity were routinely found to have photoallergic contact dermatitis.

The incidence of PACD in the general population is unknown. The available incidence data are based on positive photo–patch test results in groups of patients with presumed photosensitivity who were referred to tertiary care facilities for diagnostic photo–patch testing. In Canada, 6% of such patients who were phototested were found to have PACD in a study published in 1975. In England, 25% of tested patients were found to have positive photo–patch test responses in each year of the 1970s. The Scandinavian Multicenter Photopatch Study (1988) more recently found 274 positive photo–patch test results and 369 positive plain patch test responses in 1993 patients who were tested between 1980 and 1985. Of these, 217 patients (11%) were thought to have clinically relevant positive test responses resulting in a diagnosis of PACD. In the United States, 70 patients were tested at the Mayo Clinic during the same 5-year period. Of those tested, 38.5% and 31% had positive photo–patch test and plain patch test responses, respectively. Only 14 (20%) patients tested had clinically relevant photo–patch test reactions. In a study from New York, 187 patients were phototested; positive photo–patch test responses resulted in the diagnosis of PACD in 20 patients (11%). When these data are taken together, it would appear that the incidence of PACD in individuals with a history of a photosensitivity eruption would be approximately 10% to 20%. This rate is considerably lower than for positive test results in groups of patients patch tested because of suspected plain allergic contact dermatitis. This would suggest that the differential diagnosis of the individual with photosensitivity is more confusing and that the clinical picture of PACD is not as well defined as that for allergic contact dermatitis. More careful screening of such patients before photo–patch testing might result in a higher positive response rate but would also be likely to result in failure to correctly diagnose the condition in some individuals. A significant number of patients with a history of photosensitivity may have PACD in addition to other light-induced or light-aggravated conditions like polymorphous light eruption or connective tissue disease. The treatment of such photosensitive individuals almost invariably includes chemical sunscreening. Since some of the most common photoantigens inducing PACD are sunscreen chemicals, the optimum management of most photosensitive patients includes photo–patch testing. Failure to diagnose PACD, especially to a sunscreen agent in a photosensitive patient, could lead to an unnecessarily prolonged clinical course. Therefore it is recommended that the workup of all photosensitive patients include photo–patch testing with the standard photoallergen tray.

Photo–Patch Testing Techniques

Photo-patch testing, simply stated, is patch testing with the addition of radiation to induce formation of the photoantigen. Application of antigens and scoring criteria are the same as those described in Chapter 3 for plain patch testing. The only additional equipment that is necessary is an appropriate light source and light opaque shielding for the period after removal of the Finn chambers before readings.

All photosensitive patients should be photo–patch tested.

With very few exceptions, the most notable being diphenhydramine hydrochloride, the radiation responsible for formation of the photoantigen and clinical PACD falls within the ultraviolet A (UVA) spectrum (320 to 400 nm). The ideal light source should produce UVA radiation in a continuous spectrum (fairly uniform radiation from 320 to 400 nm) of sufficient irradiance and field size to allow irradiation of 20 to 25 antigen sites with a dose of 5 to 10 J/cm^2 within a reasonable time (about 30 minutes). The source should also produce little ultraviolet B (UVB) radiation or should be equipped with a filter to remove most of such radiation. Three to 5 mm of window glass is adequate filtration to block UVB radiation. Table 9-5 lists the most commonly available of such sources. A photometer-radiometer matched to the source is also required for proper dosimetry. Such

Table 9-5	Light Sources for Photo–Patch Testing

Ultraviolet A spectrum
  Fluorescent black lights
  Fluorescent PUVA lights
  Mercury halide lamp with a filter
  Hot quartz lamp with a filter*
  Sunlight with a filter
	Ultraviolet B spectrum
	  Fluorescent sunlamp
	  Mercury halide lamp without a filter
	  Sunlight
	  Hot quartz lamp without a filter

*Discontinuous spectrum: less desirable.
PUVA, Psoralen–ultraviolet A radiation.

source-radiometer matching is most easily accomplished by purchasing the two units from the same manufacturer. By far the most readily available source in the dermatologist's office is the unit used for delivery of photochemotherapy (psoralen UVA [PUVA]).

The dose of radiation used in photo–patch testing has varied between 1 and 10 J/cm^2 in most studies. Theoretically the largest dose that does not alone induce erythema in skin would be most likely to yield production of the photoantigen and a positive test response. Since the minimal erythema dose (MED) in the UVA range is between 20 and 60 J/cm^2, any dose that can be conveniently delivered below this level can be used, and 10 J/cm^2 has been selected more or less arbitrarily to fulfill these two criteria.

In addition to photo–patch testing, it is recommended that the patient being tested also be given graded doses of radiation in the UVB range for determination of the MED. Such testing assists in distinguishing transient and persistent light reactivity. This necessitates a UVB light source (Table 9-5).

Protocol for Photo–Patch Testing

A recommended protocol for photo–patch testing is outlined below and in Figure 9-1. This protocol should reliably diagnose PACD and also aids in the differential diagnoses of other common types of photosensitivity.

On day 1 (Figure 9-1, *A* and *B*) two sets of photoantigens are applied, one set to either side of the upper portion of the back. The antigens are applied in Finn chambers as described previously. Graded doses (8 to 10 doses) of UVB radiation are applied to previously unexposed skin sites (approximately 1 cm^2 in each area) on one buttock. These doses should include the dose of radiation that would normally correspond to the patient's MED. For a light-complexioned individual, 10, 20, 30, 40, 50, 60, 70, and 80 mJ/cm^2 would be appropriate. These doses, however, depend on the light source and photometer used. Ultraviolet A radiation at a dose to be used for photo–patch testing (usually 10 J/cm^2) is then delivered to a single site on the opposite buttock (about 1 cm^2).

On day 2 the patient returns, and the phototest sites are evaluated for erythema. The MED in the UVB range is determined as the site with minimal perceptible erythema. Whether such an MED is "normal" or "lowered" is determined by experience with the particular light source used. If there is erythema at the UVA site, this represents a definite abnormality, and titration with delivery of

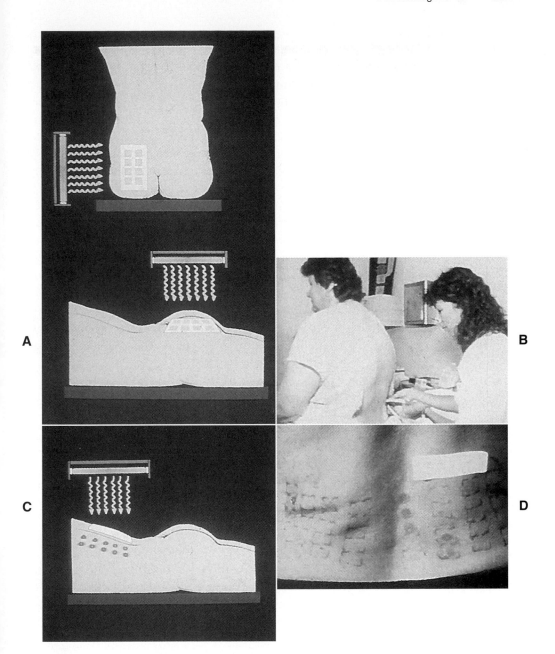

FIGURE 9-1
Suggested protocol for photobiologic testing. **A,** *Day 1:* Apply irradiation for MED. **B,** Apply two sets of antigens. *Day 2:* read MED sites. **C,** *Day 2 or 3:* Remove antigen patches. Irradiate one set of antigens. Recover antigens. **D,** *Day 4 or 5:* Read patch and photopatch tests (48 hours after irradiation). Read MED sites. *Day >5:* Perform second photopatch reading. Read MED sites.

graded doses of UVA is required to determine the proper UVA photo–patch test dose. This is done in an analogous fashion to UVB MED testing by using doses of 1, 2, 3, 4, 5, 6, 7, 8, 9, and 10 J/cm² of UVA with reading on day 3.

Assuming that a UVA radiation dose of 10 J/cm² did not elicit a response, the photo–patch test continues on day 2. Both sets of antigens are removed and marked, and readings are done at all sites for contact allergy or irritancy. One set of patches (dark control) is covered with light-opaque material, and the other set is exposed to a UVA radiation dose of 10 J/cm² (Figure 9-1, C). Then the irradiated set is also covered with light-opaque material. Gauze pads covered with aluminum foil or black felt are suitable light-opaque material. The patient returns for readings, preferably on day 4 (48 hours after irradiation) and at one later point up to a week after irradiation. Two readings are recommended and might be scheduled at 48 and 72 hours, 48 and 96 hours, or 48 hours and 1 week. If scheduling a 48-hour reading is impossible, two readings could be done at 24 and 72 hours or at 24 and 96 hours (Figure 9-1, D).

If 10 J/cm² of UVA radiation alone produced erythema, a lower dose must be used for photo–patch testing. That dose is determined by reading the MED testing (on day 3) to graded doses of UVA radiation that were applied on day 2. A dose less than the MED must be used. It is sometimes suggested that a dose of 50% of the MED should be used, but any dose that alone will not produce erythema can be used. The use of too low a dose may result in false-negative photo–patch test results. With a lowered MED in the UVA range the irradiation of patches will be on day 3. Therefore the patches are in place for 48 rather than 24 hours. There is no evidence to suggest that major differences occur between these two different testing schedules. As before, two readings should be done.

> **6-Methylcoumarin is applied 30 minutes, not 24 to 48 hours, before UVA radiation exposure. Longer application times result in false-negative photo–patch test results.**

One antigen, *6-methylcoumarin,* is not applied on day 1 with the other antigens. This agent's ability to form a photoantigen disappears rapidly after application to skin. For this reason the antigen is *applied on the day of patch irradiation* (usually day 2). It is applied in duplicate in Finn chambers for a 30-minute period before irradiation.

The photo–patch test result is read as for patch tests (outlined in Chapter 3). An area of significant controversy exists, however, in distinguishing photocontact allergy from plain contact allergy. The system used by the North American Contact Dermatitis Group is shown in Table 9-6.

Table 9-6 **Reading the Photo–Patch Test**

Diagnosis	Reading		Nonirradiated Site
	Irradiated Site		
No sensitivity	−		−
Photocontact sensitivity	+		−
Contact allergy	+		+
Photocontact and contact allergy	+ +	>	+

It is agreed that a positive response in the irradiated site and negative in the covered site is diagnostic of photoallergy. Likewise, equal positive responses in both irradiated and covered sites are diagnostic of plain contact allergy. The North American system allows for the diagnosis of both allergy and photoallergy when both sites are positive, but only when the result in the irradiated patch is significantly more positive than in the covered site. In the system used by the Scandinavian group and the Mayo Clinic group, any reaction in the covered site results in a diagnosis of plain contact allergy.

Occasionally irradiation appears to inhibit a positive patch test reaction. In such cases the nonirradiated site will be reactive, whereas the irradiated site will be negative. The pathophysiology of such an occurrence is not understood; neither are its clinical ramifications. Such a response, if clinically relevant, may be significant.

As with plain patch testing, false-positive and false-negative results can occur in photo–patch testing. One particularly common false-positive or photoirritant response is to the phenothiazine agents in the tray (chlorpromazine and promethazine), which is discussed in detail in those antigen sections of this chapter.

Some antigens produce an immediate photoirritant response. Erythema is noted at the completion of the irradiation period. This is not usually clinically relevant and may be disregarded.

In addition to the photoallergens in the tray, patients can be tested to their own products, particularly to sunscreens and fragrance-containing cosmetics. Industrial cleansers and the like, as well as personal care cleansers that may be the source for antibacterial agents, must be diluted approximately as detailed in Chapter 3 for such testing.

Chronic Actinic Dermatitis: Persistent Light Reactions

As with plain contact dermatitis, avoidance of contact with the photoallergen in a patient with PACD usually results in clearing of the dermatitis and the photosensitivity. Occasionally, however, the patient continues to be photosensitive, that is, he or she continues to react to light with the development of dermatitis. Such patients were first observed with the antibacterial photoallergens and were called *persistent light reactors.* In contrast, patients whose conditions clear once the photoallergen is removed were called *transient light reactors.*

Occasionally, persistent photosensitivity remained localized to the distribution of the original photoallergen exposure. This was called a *localized persistent light reaction* and was seen with the antibacterial bithionol. In such patients it was postulated that the sensitivity was related to persistence of allergen at the sites of initial exposure. In these individuals exposure of previously uninvolved skin to UV radiation produced normal reactions (normal MED in the UVB and UVA ranges). Photo–patch testing (UVA and allergen), of course, produced a positive response.

Other patients, however, developed a generalized photosensitivity in the absence of continued antigen exposure. Most notable were patients who were photoallergic to the antibacterials tetrachlorosalicylanilide (TCSA) and tribromosalicylanilide (TBS) and, more recently, to the fragrance musk ambrette

(Figure 9-2). In these individuals exposure of previously uninvolved skin to irradiation without allergen resulted in abnormal reactivity. This resulted in a lowered MED in the UVB range (possibly in the UVA and visible ranges). These responses were different both quantitatively and qualitatively from sunburn or MED erythema. On clinical and histologic examination the reactions were eczematous. The responses represented a reproduction of the clinical eruption without antigen. This type of response is more difficult to explain pathophysiologically than the localized persistent light reactions. Not only has skin not previously exposed to light or antigen developed sensitivity, but also the spectrum has shifted from UVA into the UVB range. It has been suggested that the original photoallergic reaction (UVA radiation plus allergen) has resulted in the development of an endogenous photoallergen, probably an altered carrier protein, with absorption and activation in the UVB range. Only certain photoallergens are apparently capable of inducing such sensitivity. This includes a number of the antibacterial halogenated phenols, phenothiazines, and musk ambrette.

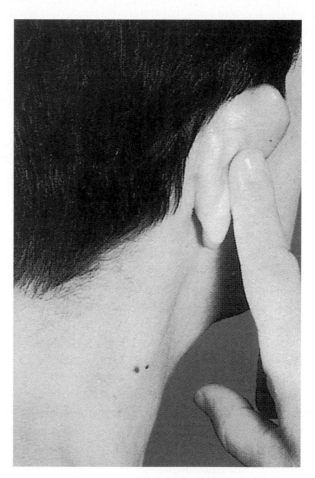

FIGURE 9-2
Chronic actinic dermatitis involving the neck but sparing the postauricular area.

Persistent light reactivity has most frequently been reported to be due to antibacterial salicylanilides and the fragrance musk ambrette.

Although the severity of photosensitivity in patients with persistent light reaction varies greatly, many patients have been severely debilitated. Such individuals reacted adversely to minimal sun exposure (less than 1 minute of natural exposure) and were even believed to be reacting to indoor fluorescent lighting. The eczematous eruption became chronic and spread to involve non–sun-exposed areas, sometimes eventuating in generalized erythroderma. Histologic study occasionally revealed an atypical infiltrate, leading to the misdiagnosis of mycosis fungoides. Such patients were said to have *actinic reticuloid.* Most such patients were older men. Patients of similar age and sex with a similar disseminated photosensitive eczematous response have also been reported under the terms *photosensitive eczema, eczematous polymorphous light eruption,* and *photosensitivity dermatitis.* The photobiologic criteria for diagnosis of these various conditions are listed in Table 9-7. All of these patients have in common a persistent eczematous clinical eruption of sun-exposed skin with possible extension to non–sun-exposed areas, sensitivity to UVB radiation (with possible sensitivity to UVA and visible radiation), and chronic eczematous changes on skin biopsy with or without atypical infiltrate. It has been noted that patients may develop and/or lose criteria for differentiating these various diagnoses. Therefore it has been suggested that all such patients represent variations of a single process and that they all be grouped under the diagnosis chronic actinic dermatitis. Patients with chronic actinic dermatitis may have positive photo–patch test responses. They may also have multiple positive plain patch test reactions to airborne or industrially relevant antigens like chrysanthemum and dichromates. Chronic actinic dermatitis is also reported to occur without other apparent cause in human immunodeficiency virus–positive patients. Photobiologic testing in these individuals reveals a lowered MED to UVB radiation. The test site is eczematous on clinical and histologic examination.

Table 9-7 — Chronic Actinic Dermatitis

Original Terminology	Abnormal Reactivity			Photo–Patch Test	Atypical Histology
	UVB	UVA	Visible		
Actinic reticuloid	+	+/–	+/–	+/–	+
Photosensitive dermatitis	+	+/–	–	+/–	–
Photosensitive eczema	+	–	–	–	–
Persistent light reaction	+	+/–	–	+	–
Eczematous PMLE	+	+/–	–	–	–

PMLE, Polymorphous light eruption; *UVA,* ultraviolet A radiation; *UVB,* ultraviolet B radiation.

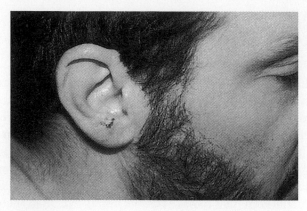

FIGURE 9-3
Photoallergic contact dermatitis from benzophenone in sunscreens.

Sunscreen Agents

In the decades of the 1970s and 1980s people in the United States, Europe, and Australia began to increase their usage of sunscreens as they were educated to the dangers of sun exposure. This has led to increased exposure to active ingredients in these products. Therefore it is not surprising that such agents induce contact allergy, and because such ingredients by definition absorb UV radiation, it is not surprising that they also induce PACD. The incidence of these reactions in the sunscreen-using population is unknown, but it is probably very low. The incidence of such reactions in groups of patients with photosensitivity, however, is high. Sunscreen components were the most common group of agents producing relevant photo–patch test reactions in a New York photo–patch test series and in a series of 250 patients tested by the North American Contact Dermatitis Group from 1992 to 1998. Sunscreen reactions were less frequent than antimicrobials and fragrances reactions in the Mayo Clinic and Scandinavian studies (Figure 9-3).

p-AMINOBENZOIC ACID
Definition

p-Aminobenzoic acid (PABA) was the first chemical agent to be used extensively in sunscreens sold in the United States. The recommended photo–patch test concentration is 5% in alcohol, although 5% in petrolatum is sometimes used. It was the most common sensitizer in the sunscreen group of photoallergens in the Scandinavian photo–patch test study. In that study 2% of all patients were reported to have positive photo–patch test responses, and 2% were reported to have positive plain contact patch test reactions to this antigen. In a later series of patients tested by the North American Contact Dermatitis Group, 1.2% of the patients tested were reported to have a positive photo–patch test, and 3.2% were reported to have positive plain patch tests. In that study done between 1992 and 1998, this allergen was the least common photoallergen of the sunscreen agents giving positive responses.

Clinical Aspects

PABA is an excellent absorber of radiation in the UVB range. Recognition of this fact in the 1950s led to its being used as the first chemical sunscreen in the 1960s. It was widely used and was a component of most sunscreens marketed in the 1960s and 1970s. One major drawback was its potential to stain clothing. Contact and photocontact dermatitis has been infrequently ascribed to this agent. The perception that "PABA allergy" was a common occurrence led to a consumer misconception that any adverse response of the skin when sunscreen was used was due to such PABA allergy. This has led to the manufacture and marketing of many PABA-free sunscreens. PABA is now used only occasionally in sunscreen products in the United States.

In addition to products marketed as sunscreens, PABA may also be used in cosmetics such as moisturizers and emollients, lipsticks and lip balms, and shampoos and other hair products, as well as being used as an oral vitamin supplement. The latter, however, has not been reported to induce a systemic contact dermatitis or photosensitivity.

Most photocontact and contact allergy to PABA results in a dermatitis of sun-exposed areas, since application of sunscreen products are usually confined to those areas. If the patient is photoallergic but not contact allergic to PABA, he or she does not react each time the agent is applied but reacts only when the dose of radiation has been sufficient to produce the photoallergen. This lack of response on each application may convince the patient that the sunscreen is not the problem.

In addition, photoallergy to PABA may complicate or be confused with other types of photosensitivity, particularly polymorphous light eruption.

In all likelihood, patients with contact and photocontact allergies to PABA do not routinely seek medical attention, since an adverse reaction leads to a change to a PABA-free sunscreen by well-educated consumers.

> **Patients who are photoallergic to PABA or other photoantigens do not react each time the antigen is applied but react only when radiation is also present in sufficient dose.**

Patients who are allergic or photoallergic to PABA may also react to the other PABA-derivative sunscreens and to the chemically related systemic and topical agents listed in Table 9-8.

Although PABA is tested at 5% concentration in alcohol in the North American Contact Dermatitis Group tray, it has also been tested at concentrations varying from 1% to 10% in both alcohol and petrolatum. There are reports of false-negative reactions when the petrolatum vehicle is used.

Table 9-8

Chemicals That May Cause Dermatitis in Patients Who Are Allergic or Photoallergic to PABA and PABA-Derivative Sunscreens

Class	Chemical
Sunscreens	Para-aminobenzoic acid (PABA)
	Amyl dimethyl PABA (padimate A)
	Octyl dimethyl PABA (padimate O)
	Glycerol PABA
Diuretic	Hydrochlorothiazide (Hydrodiuril)
Antidiabetic agent	Sulfonylureas (tolbutamide)
Hair dye	p-Phenylenediamine
Anesthetic	Benzocaine
Antiinfective	p-Aminosalicylic acid
Cardiac drug	Procaine (procainamide)

EXPOSURE LIST   ▶   *p*-AMINOBENZOIC ACID

Synonyms and Other Names

Aminobenzoic acid   Papcidium
PAB   Vitamin H
PABA

Uses

PABA is found primarily in creams, lotions, sprays, and sticks used as sunscreens. It may also be found in the following:
1. Moisturizers
2. Cosmetics
3. Shampoos and other hair care products
4. Nail polish
5. Lipsticks and lip balms
6. Oral vitamin supplements

Prevention

Patients may be allergic or photoallergic to PABA. If photoallergic, they may not react to PABA alone but only with sun exposure. In either case, contact with this agent and with related chemicals or PABA derivatives should be avoided. This includes *padimate A* (amyl dimethyl PABA), *padimate O* (octyl dimethyl PABA), and *glycerol PABA*. To avoid these chemicals, the labels of all sun-protective agents and the other products previously listed must be read, and agents with oxybenzone, sulisobenzone, cinnamates, dibenzoylmethane, or salicylates may be substituted. Many such "PABA-free" products are available. In addition, patients should be instructed to make all their health care providers aware that a reaction to some medications, including thiazide diuretics, sulfonylurea antidiabetic agents, *p*-aminosalicylic acid, procainamide (procaine), and benzocaine, may develop. Allergic individuals should be told that they may also react to the *p*-phenylenediamine present in permanent hair dyes.

AMYL DIMETHYL PABA

Definition

Amyl *N*-dimethyl *p*-aminobenzoate (amyl dimethyl *p*-aminobenzoic acid [PABA], padimate A) is a PABA ester. It is rarely used in sunscreens today in the United States. This chemical is tested at 5% concentration in petrolatum. In groups of photosensitive patients tested in the United States, 3% of patients had positive photo–patch test responses to this antigen.

Clinical Aspects

Amyl dimethyl PABA was one of three PABA derivatives developed and marketed as sunscreening agents. It was soon noted to produce an immediate type of phototoxicity. This resulted in burning and stinging on exposure to light. Although it is approved as safe and effective in the 1978 Food and Drug Administration (FDA) monograph on sunscreens, it is almost never used in sunscreens marketed in the United States today. Patients who are sensitive to this agent may also react to PABA and other PABA derivatives and to the topical and systemic agents listed in Table 9-8.

EXPOSURE LIST ▸ **AMYL DIMETHYL PABA**

Synonyms and Other Names

Amyl *N*-dimethylaminobenzoate
Escalol 506
Isoamyl *N*-dimethylaminobenzoate
Isoamyl *N*-dimethyl PABA

Padimate A
Pentyl dimethyl PABA
Spectraban

Uses

The agent amyl dimethyl PABA is used primarily in creams, lotions, sprays, and sticks sold as sunscreens. It may also be found in the following products:
1. Moisturizers
2. Cosmetics
3. Shampoos and other hair care products
4. Nail polish
5. Lipsticks and lip balms

Prevention

Patients may be allergic or photoallergic to amyl dimethyl PABA. If photoallergic, they may not react to amyl dimethyl PABA alone but only with light exposure. In either case they should avoid contact with this agent and with related chemicals or PABA derivatives. This includes PABA, *padimate O* (octyl dimethyl PABA), and *glycerol PABA*. To avoid these chemicals, allergic persons must read the labels of all sun-protective agents and the other products previously listed and substitute these agents with oxybenzone, sulisobenzone, cinnamates, dibenzoylmethane, or salicylates. Many such "PABA-free" products are available. In addition, allergic patients should be instructed to make all their health care providers aware that they may develop a reaction from some medications, including thiazide diuretics, sulfonylurea antidiabetic agents, *p*-aminosalicylic acid, procainamide (procaine), and benzocaine. Such patients must be made aware that they may also react to the *p*-phenylenediamine present in permanent hair dyes.

May be duplicated for use in clinical practice. From Marks JG Jr, Elsner P, DeLeo VA: *Contact and occupational dermatology,* ed 3, St Louis, 2002, Mosby.

OCTYL DIMETHYL PABA

Definition

Octyl dimethyl PABA (padimate O) is a PABA derivative that is used primarily as a sunscreen. It is tested at a concentration of 5% in petrolatum. The Scandinavian multicenter photo–patch test study found that 2.5% of its photosensitive patients were contact allergic to this agent and none were photoallergic (2% concentration tested). The North American Contact Dermatitis Group found that 1.6% of patients were photoallergic to this agent and 3.6% of patients were contact allergic.

Clinical Aspects

Octyl dimethyl PABA is a PABA derivative that is used as a sunscreening agent. Of the PABA group, it is the most commonly used agent in sunscreens marketed in the United States. It may also be found in cosmetics for skin, hair, and nails, such as moisturizers, lipsticks, and lip balms. Unlike PABA, octyl dimethyl PABA is not water soluble and binds to the stratum corneum. It appears to be a rare sensitizer but has been reported to cause both contact and photocontact dermatitis. The resultant dermatitis is usually in a photodistribution, even in cases of contact rather than photocontact dermatitis, because sunscreen usage is commonly limited to sun-exposed areas. Patients who are photoallergic may fail to recognize the origin of their problem, since application of the chemical without sufficient radiation does not result in lesion development.

EXPOSURE LIST ▶ **OCTYL DIMETHYL PABA**

Synonyms and Other Names

Escalol 507

2-Ethylhexyl-*p*-dimethylaminobenzoate

Octyl dimethylaminobenzoate

Padimate O

Uses

This agent is used primarily in creams, lotions, sprays, and sticks used as sunscreens. It may also be found in the following products:

1. Moisturizers
2. Cosmetics
3. Shampoos and other hair care products
4. Nail polish
5. Lipsticks and lip balms

Prevention

Patients may be allergic or photoallergic to octyl dimethyl PABA. If photoallergic, they may not react to padimate O alone but only with light exposure. In either case, they should avoid contact with this agent and with related PABA derivatives. This includes PABA, *padimate A* (amyl dimethyl PABA), and *glycerol PABA*. To avoid these chemicals, patients must be instructed to read the labels of all sun-protective agents as well as the other products listed previously, and substitute these agents with oxybenzone, sulisobenzone, cinnamates, dibenzoylmethane, or salicylates. Many such "PABA-free" products are available.

Allergic individuals should be instructed to make all their health care providers aware that they may have reactions to some medications, including thiazide diuretics, sulfonylurea antidiabetic agents, *p*-aminosalicylic acid, procainamide (procaine), and benzocaine. Such patients must be made aware that they may also react to the *p*-phenylenediamine that is present in permanent hair dyes.

May be duplicated for use in clinical practice. From Marks JG Jr, Elsner P, DeLeo VA: *Contact and occupational dermatology,* ed 3, St Louis, 2002, Mosby.

Octyl dimethyl PABA (padimate O) is the most frequently used PABA-group sunscreen agent in the United States.

Patients who are allergic or photoallergic to octyl dimethyl PABA may also react adversely to PABA- and PABA-derivative–containing sunscreens and to the topical and systemic agents listed in Table 9-8. There is a single reported case of possible cross-sensitization or cosensitization between cinoxate and octyl dimethyl PABA.

OCTYL METHOXYCINNAMATE
Definition
Octyl methoxycinnamate is a UVB absorber that is commonly used in sunscreens in the United States. It is tested at 7.5% concentration in petrolatum. It is a low-level sensitizer accounting for one positive photo–patch test response in 108 patients in an Italian study and one positive patch test response and one positive photo–patch test response in 280 patients tested in London. Of the 250 patients tested by the North American Contact Dermatitis Group, none were found to be allergic or photoallergic to this agent.

Clinical Aspects
The cinnamates are a group of chemically related substances that are used as fragrances and flavorings and less frequently as sunscreens. Two of the UV-absorbing

---

EXPOSURE LIST ▶ **OCTYL METHOXYCINNAMATE**

Synonyms and Other Names

2-Ethylhexyl methoxycinnamate

Givauden

3-(4-Methoxyphenyl)-2-propenoic acid, 2-ethylhexyl ester

Parsol MCX

Uses

Octyl methoxycinnamate is used primarily in creams, lotions, sprays, and sticks used as sunscreens. It may also be found in the following products:

1. Moisturizers
2. Cosmetics
3. Shampoos and other hair care products
4. Nail polish
5. Lipsticks and lip balms

Prevention

Labels of all sunscreens and the agents listed previously should be examined carefully, and patients should be made aware that reactions may occur only with sun exposure and therefore a reaction may not occur each time the product is used. In addition to the previously listed names, reactions may also occur to fragrances and flavoring agents and to other sunscreen agents that end in the word "cinnamate." Allergic patients may need to avoid fragranced cosmetics and certain toothpastes and mouthwashes to prevent dermatitis.

May be duplicated for use in clinical practice. From Marks JG Jr, Elsner P, DeLeo VA: *Contact and occupational dermatology,* ed 3, St Louis, 2002, Mosby.

agents in this group, 2-ethoxyethyl-*p*-methoxy-cinnamate (cinoxate) and octyl-*p*-methoxycinnamate (Parsol MCX), are approved by the FDA for usage as sunscreens. Octyl methoxycinnamate is being used in increasing numbers of sunscreen products in the United States. It appears to be a very low-level sensitizer.

Patients who are allergic to this sunscreening ingredient may react adversely to flavorings and fragrances of the cinnamate group.

OCTYL SALICYLATE

Definition

Octyl salicylate is one of four salicylates approved for usage as UV-absorbing chemicals in sunscreen products in the United States. Only two, octyl salicylate and homosalate, are used presently. Although not previously reported to cause sensitization, octyl salicylate is gaining increased usage in the United States and therefore is included in the photoallergen tray. It is tested at a concentration of 5% in petrolatum.

> **Four salicylates are approved for usage in over-the-counter sunscreens in the United States. Only two, octyl salicylate and homosalate, are used.**

Clinical Aspects

Octyl salicylate is a UV-absorbing salicylate that is widely used in sunscreens. It has not been reported to cause contact or photocontact dermatitis, but because of

---

EXPOSURE LIST ▶ **OCTYL SALICYLATE**

Synonyms and Other Names
Dermablock OS
2-Ethylhexyl 2-hydroxybenzoate
2-Ethylhexyl Salicylate
Sunarome WNO

Uses
Octyl salicylate is found primarily in creams, lotions, sprays, and sticks used as sunscreens. It may also be found in the following:
1. Moisturizers
2. Cosmetics
3. Shampoos and other hair care products
4. Nail polish
5. Lipsticks and lip balms

Prevention
Patients may be allergic or photoallergic to octyl salicylate. If photoallergic, they may not react to the agent alone but only with sun exposure. In either case, contact with this agent and with related chemicals should be avoided. This includes homosalate. To avoid these chemicals, the labels of all sun-protective agents and the other products listed previously must be read, and agents with oxybenzone, sulisobenzone, cinnamates, dibenzoylmethane, or PABA derivatives should be substituted.

Patients should be instructed to make all their health care providers aware that, although it is unlikely, a reaction to some medications, including aspirin, methyl salicylate, and tartrazine dye may develop.

May be duplicated for use in clinical practice. From Marks JG Jr, Elsner P, DeLeo VA: *Contact and occupational dermatology,* ed 3, St Louis, 2002, Mosby.

widespread usage, such reactions may occur. The salicylates are a large group of chemically related compounds including antiinflammatory agents like aspirin and flavoring agents like methyl salicylate (oil of wintergreen) and the related dye tartrazine (FD & C Yellow Dye No. 5). Cross-reaction to these agents in patients sensitized to the UV-absorbing salicylates are theoretically possible but have not been reported.

OXYBENZONE

Definition

Oxybenzone (2-hydroxy-4-methoxybenzophenone) is a UV-absorbing agent that is used extensively in commercially available sunscreens. It is tested at 3% concentration in petrolatum. It produced positive reactions in 9.5% of 187 photosensitive patients tested in the New York study (1%, contact; 5.3%, photocontact; 3.2%, both contact and photocontact); 1.5% (photocontact) of patients tested at the Mayo Clinic; and 1% (0.9%, photocontact; 0.1%, contact) of patients tested in Scandinavia. In the most recent study done by the North American Contact Dermatitis Group, 4.8% of patients were found to be photoallergic to this agent, and 6.4% were found to be contact allergic.

Clinical Aspects

Oxybenzone is one of the most commonly used active ingredient in sunscreens marketed in the United States today. It is used in single- and multiple-agent products and in PABA-free and PABA-containing products. It also appears to be the most frequently used UV-absorbing agent included in nonsunscreen cosmetics like moisturizers and agents advertised for their antiaging effects.

Benzophenones are a group of 12 diphenylketones that are used as UV absorbers in industrial coatings and sunscreens. They are also used as preservatives, since some members of this group, especially benzophenone 2, have excellent antimicrobial activity.

> **Oxybenzone is one of the most commonly used sunscreening agents in the United States.**

Photocontact allergy and contact allergy to these agents have only recently been recognized and are probably rare. Even so, with such extensive usage oxybenzone is certainly one of the most common agents responsible for PACD today.

Cross-sensitization among agents in the benzophenone group has been reported.

Two NSAID agents of the arylpropionic group, ketoprofen and tiaprofenic acid, and the cholesterol-lowering agent fenofibrate contain a benzophenone moiety. All have been reported to cause photoallergy when taken systemically. Ketoprofen (not available in the United States) has been reported to produce photoallergic contact dermatitis when used topically. Oxybenzone has been reported to cross-react with these other agents; sulisobenzone, however, has not shown the same reactivity.

<table>
<tr><td colspan="2">EXPOSURE LIST ▷ OXYBENZONE</td></tr>
</table>

Synonyms and Other Names

Benzophenone-3   2-Hydroxy-4-methoxybenzophenone
Eusolex 4360   Uvinul M-40

Uses

Oxybenzone is used primarily in creams, lotions, sprays, and sticks used as sunscreens. It may also be found in the following products:
1. Moisturizers
2. Cosmetics
3. Shampoos and other hair care products
4. Nail polish
5. Lipsticks and lip balms

Prevention

Patients may be allergic to photoallergic to oxybenzone. If photoallergic, they may not react to oxybenzone alone but only on light exposure. In either case, they should avoid contact with this agent. Such patients may also react adversely to other benzophenones and therefore should avoid them as well. To avoid these chemicals, patients must be instructed to read the labels of all sunscreen products and the products listed previously to look for the names listed as well as sulisobenzone and benzophenone with a number designation (e.g., benzophenone 2). Allergic patients may use sunscreens composed of PABA, padimate, cinnamate, salicylates, and dibenzoylmethane.

   Patients who are allergic or photoallergic to oxybenzone should avoid the nonsteroidal antiinflammatory agents (NSAIDs) ketoprofen and tiaprofenic acid and the cholesterol-lowering agent fenofibrate, all of which contain a benzophenone moiety.

May be duplicated for use in clinical practice. From Marks JG Jr, Elsner P, DeLeo VA: *Contact and occupational dermatology,* ed 3, St Louis, 2002, Mosby.

SULISOBENZONE

Definition

Sulisobenzone (2-hydroxy-4-methoxybenzophenone-5-sulfonic acid) is a UV-absorbing agent that is used in commercially available sunscreens. It is tested at 10% concentration in petrolatum. This antigen produced positive photo–patch test results in 3% of patients tested in the Mayo Clinic series. In the North American Contact Dermatitis Group study, 3.25% of patients tested were found to be photoallergic to this agent, and 0.8% were found to be contact allergic.

Clinical Aspects

Benzophenones are a group of UV-absorbing diphenylketones originally used as a coating for materials in industry to protect from discoloration. Twelve benzophenones are used in the United States and are designated as benzophenones 1 through 12. Sulisobenzone is one of three benzophenones approved for use in sunscreens in the United States and was the first to achieve significant usage. It was used in some of the original, single-agent PABA-free sunscreens that were manufactured. In recent years its usage has decreased while the usage of oxybenzone has increased greatly.

   Sulisobenzone is an infrequently reported contact and photocontact sensitizer.

EXPOSURE LIST ➤ **SULISOBENZONE**

Synonyms and Other Names

Benzophenone 4

5-Benzoyl-4-hydroxy-2-methoxybenzene-sulfonic acid

2 Hydroxy-4-methoxybenzophenone-5-sulfonic acid

Spectra-Sorb UV 284

Uval

Uvistat 1121

Uses

Sulisobenzone is used primarily in creams, lotions, sprays, and sticks used as sunscreens. It may also be found in the following products:

1. Moisturizers
2. Cosmetics
3. Shampoos and other hair care products
4. Nail polish
5. Lipsticks and lip balms

Prevention

Patients may be allergic or photoallergic to sulisobenzone. If photoallergic, they may not react to sulisobenzone but only on light exposure. In either case, they should avoid contact with this agent. Such patients may also react adversely to other benzophenones and should therefore be instructed to avoid them as well. To avoid these chemicals, patients must be instructed to read the labels of all sunscreen products and the products previously listed to look for the names listed as well as for oxybenzone and benzophenone with a number designation (e.g., benzophenone 2). Allergic individuals may use sunscreens composed of PABA, padimate, cinnamate, salicylates, and dibenzoylmethanes.

May be duplicated for use in clinical practice. From Marks JG Jr, Elsner P, DeLeo VA: *Contact and occupational dermatology,* ed 3, St Louis, 2002, Mosby.

It has been reported to be associated with cross-sensitization to oxybenzone and benzophenone 2, which is frequently used as a cosmetic preservative.

> **Benzophenones are UV-absorbing chemicals that are used as sunscreens and as preservatives and industrial coatings.**

Fragrances

A number of fragrance ingredients have been associated with photoallergic contact dermatitis. Two of these appear to cause significant problems—musk ambrette and 6-methylcoumarin. The former was used in men's aftershave and cologne and has caused severe, persistent reactions; the latter was used as the fragrance in suntanning lotion and caused severe but transient reactions. A third agent, sandalwood oil, has infrequently been reported to induce photosensitization.

> **The most common fragrance photoallergens are 6-methylcoumarin and musk ambrette.**

6-METHYLCOUMARIN

Definition

6-Methylcoumarin is a synthetic fragrance chemically related to the psoralens. It is tested at a concentration of 1% in alcohol. Unlike all the other photoantigens, this antigen is applied 30 minutes, not 24 to 48 hours, before irradiation. It has produced positive photo–patch test reactions in 0.2% of photosensitive patients tested in Scandinavia and 0.5% of patients tested in New York. In contrast, 7% of patients tested at the Mayo Clinic were found to be photoallergic to this antigen. Only one patient (0.05%) with a positive plain contact reaction to the antigen was found in the three studies.

Clinical Aspects

6-Methylcoumarin is a synthetic fragrance ingredient with a fruity coconut odor. It is used in cosmetics and in the early 1980s was used as a fragrance ingredient in suntanning lotion. Despite premarketing testing that failed to reveal photosensitization, a large number of patients developed a photoallergic contact dermatitis to the suntanning lotion. Such reactions were extensive and severe and required hospitalization in some patients. The reactions had features of both phototoxicity and photoallergy. Discovering the photoallergen in the lotion was not immediately achieved by routine photo–patch testing until it was discovered that 6-methylcoumarin rapidly becomes inactive as a photoallergen on application to skin. False-negative results occur when the agent is applied for 24 to 48 hours before irradiation. For this reason it is recommended that the antigen be applied in duplicate 30 minutes before irradiation.

> **6-Methylcoumarin caused photoallergic contact dermatitis when it was used as a fragrance ingredient in sunscreen products.**

The International Fragrance Association has recommended that this agent no longer be used in personal care products. Although it is no longer used in suntanning products, it may still be found in other cosmetic products, and occasional reports of problems with old, outdated suntanning lotions manufactured in the early 1980s still appear.

> **When photo–patch testing with 6-methylcoumarin, one must apply the antigen to the skin for no longer than 30 minutes before UVA exposure. Application for 24 to 48 hours may lead to false-negative photo–patch test results.**

Some investigators test at a higher concentration of 5% in alcohol or petrolatum.

MUSK AMBRETTE

Definition

Musk ambrette (2-methoxy-3,5-dinitro-4-methyl-*tert*-butylbenzone) is a synthetic fragrance fixative with a potent floral odor that is used primarily in cosmetics for men. It is tested at 1% concentration in petrolatum. In the 1980s it was the most commonly reported topical photoantigen. This antigen produced positive photo–patch test responses in 2.8% of photosensitive patients tested in Scandinavia, 12.9% at the Mayo Clinic, and 4.8% in New York. It produced positive contact patch test results in 0.6% and 0.5% of patients in the Scandinavian and New York studies, respectively. In the North American Contact Dermatitis Group study done in the 1990s, years after the removal of this fragrance from marketed products in the United States, 2.4% of patients with photosensitivity were found to be photoallergic to this allergen, and 1.2% were found to be contact allergic to it.

Clinical Aspects

Natural musks are obtained from the scent glands of animals and some plants. These agents have been used in fragrances as fixatives or enhancers for decades. Synthesis of these fragrance ingredients has allowed for less expensive and therefore more extensive usage. Musk ambrette is one such agent. In the 1970s and 1980s it was used in quantities greater than 50 tons per year in the United States alone. Concentrations as high as 15% were used, and aftershaves were the most common type of product containing this agent. The first cases of photosensitivity to this agent were reported in the late 1970s. Since that time a great deal of literature on the frequency of response and mechanisms of pathophysiology has appeared. Musk ambrette was certainly the most frequently encountered topical photoantigen of the 1980s. In addition to inducing transient light reactions, it also induced many cases of severely debilitating, persistent light reactions (chronic actinic dermatitis). These latter patients reacted to UV radiation long after discontinuation of antigen exposure. The area of involvement with dermatitis frequently extended to non–sun-exposed areas and erythroderma.

EXPOSURE LIST ▷ **MUSK AMBRETTE**

Synonyms and Other Names
2,2-Methoxy-3,5-dinitro-4-methyl-*tert*-butylbenzone

Uses
Musk ambrette is a fragrance ingredient of aftershaves, colognes, and other cosmetics for men.

Prevention
All fragranced products should be avoided, especially but not only aftershaves and colognes. Household products and cosmetics used by close family members should also be fragrance-free.

───────

May be duplicated for use in clinical practice. From Marks JG Jr, Elsner P, DeLeo VA: *Contact and occupational dermatology,* ed 3, St Louis, 2002, Mosby.

> **Musk ambrette in men's colognes was the most frequent cause of photoallergic contact dermatitis in the 1980s.**

Patients with transient light reactions frequently had a patchy distribution of dermatitis on the face and neck with many spared areas. This was probably due to the usage pattern of the agent in aftershave.

The International Fragrance Association has recommended that musk ambrette not be used in cosmetics and toiletries that come into contact with skin. For other applications the Association recommends a concentration of less than 4%. Although the exact current usage pattern in the United States and Europe is unknown, usage is markedly decreased but musk ambrette may still be present in a number of cosmetic products.

Other investigators have recommended testing at a higher concentration of 5% in petrolatum or alcohol.

SANDALWOOD OIL

Definition

Sandalwood oil is an essential oil that is used as a fragrance ingredient in cosmetics. It is tested "as is." It produced a single positive photo–patch test result in a series of 187 photosensitive patients tested in New York.

Clinical Aspects

Sandalwood oil (oil of Santal) is an essential oil obtained from the heartwood of *Santalum album,* a small evergreen that is native to India and Malaysia. The natural oil contains santal and santalene, among other ingredients. Commercial sandalwood oil is composed of the natural and synthetic oil of Santal as well as additives, including synthetic geranium, geranium bourbon, cedar wood oil, and patchouli oil. Commercial sandalwood oil has a woodsy aroma (said to be "masculine") and is used primarily in men's perfumes, aftershaves, and soaps. It has

---

EXPOSURE LIST ▶ **SANDALWOOD OIL**

Synonyms and Other Uses
Arheol
East Indian sandalwood oil
Oil of Santal

Uses
Sandalwood oil is used as a fragrance in the following products:
1. Soaps
2. Aftershaves
3. Cologne
4. Cosmetics

Prevention
Patients who are photoallergic or allergic to a fragrance product should be instructed to use only fragrance-free cosmetics and personal care products.

May be duplicated for use in clinical practice. From Marks JG Jr, Elsner P, DeLeo VA: *Contact and occupational dermatology,* ed 3, St Louis, 2002, Mosby.

---

been reported to cause plain allergic contact dermatitis, photocontact dermatitis, and persistent light reaction. In one well-documented case the actual photoantigen in a case of sandalwood oil photoallergy was found to be synthetic geranium and geranium bourbon.

Sandalwood oil is also used as an incense and fumigant.

Antibacterial Agents

The first major epidemic of PACD occurred in the military during World War II when topical sulfonamides were used to treat battlefield wounds. It was not until 1960 that significant numbers of the general population were affected with this condition. Within 3 years (1960 to 1962), over 10,000 individuals were thought to have developed PACD to another antibacterial agent, tetrachlorosalicylanilide (TCSA). TCSA is a halogenated phenol that was used extensively in a bar soap in England and to a lesser extent in the United States. Once it was recognized for its photosensitizing potential, it was removed from the market.

> **Tetrachlorosalicylanilide (TCSA), which was used in bar soaps, induced an epidemic of photoallergic contact dermatitis in the 1960s.**

A number of related chemicals have since been used as antibacterials in soaps, deodorants, shampoos, and cosmetics. Some of these have likewise been implicated in producing PACD. The more highly sensitizing agents like tribromosalicylanilide (TBS) have been removed from consumer products in the extensive usage as a surgical-scrub cleanser. It is used as a preoperative scrub for operating room personnel but is also used for hand washing in many other health care settings. It is used as a cleanser of the operative site in both skin and mucosa. It is used to cleanse burns and trauma sites and used as a mouthwash in treatment of periodontal disease and in gynecologic and urologic procedures. Chlorhexidine has been used in eyedrops, contact lens care products, toothpaste, and mouthwash and as a preservative in various cosmetics, personal care products, and topical medications.

The three salts of chlorhexidine that are used include the digluconate (gluconate), diacetate (acetate), and dihydrochloride. The first two are more frequently used in the United States. These agents are rarely sensitizing (plain and photo). When tested at 1% concentration, these agents may induce irritancy. Testing must be done in an aqueous solution, since petrolatum tends to yield false-negative plain contact and photo–patch test results. Cross-reactions between the two salts commonly occur. Cross-reactivity with the other halogenated phenols is not reported.

EXPOSURE LIST ▶ CHLORHEXIDINE

Synonyms and Other Names

Chlorhexidien diacetate (acetate)
Chlorhexidine digluconate (gluconate)
Chlorhexidine dihydrochloride
Diacetate
   Chlorasept 2000
   Nolvasan
Digluconate
   Corsodyl
   Hibiclens

Hibidil
Hibiscrub
Hibitane
Plac Out
Plurexid
Rotersept
Dihydrochloride
   Lisium

Uses

Chlorhexidine is used primarily as an antibacterial cleanser in the medical setting. It is also used as a preservative in cosmetics and person care products and has the following applications:

1. Surgical-scrub cleanser
2. Hand cleanser (liquid)
3. Toothpaste, mouthwash, gum treatment
4. Eyedrops, contact lens care products
5. Wound cleanser
6. Cosmetics and personal care products

Prevention

Patients allergic or photoallergic to chlorhexidine should be instructed to avoid all the chemically related chlorhexidines listed previously by carefully reading the labels of liquid hand cleaners and the other products listed. In addition, such individuals should make all their health care workers aware of their allergy, because chlorhexidine frequently is used to cleanse the skin and internal sites during minor and major surgical and dental procedures.

DICHLOROPHEN(E)

Definition

Dichlorophen(e) (2,2-methylenebis[4-chlorophenol]) is a phenolic antimicrobial that is used as a bactericide and fungicide in many personal care cleansers and cosmetics. It is tested at a concentration of 1% in petrolatum. Dichlorophen induced positive photo–patch test reactions in 2 of 70 photosensitive patients tested in the Mayo Clinic series and 2 of 187 patients tested in the New York study.

EXPOSURE LIST	DICHLOROPHEN(E)

Synonyms and Other Names

Anthiphen	Hyosan
Cuniphen	Parabis
Dicestal	Teniathane
Didroxane	Teniatol
2,2-Dihydroxydiphenylmethane	Wespuril
G-4 (Compound G4)	

Uses

This agent is used as an antiinfective, an antibacterial, and a preservative in the following personal care products:
1. Shampoos
2. Soaps and cleansers
3. Dentifrices, toothpaste, and mouthwashes
4. Deodorants
5. Foot powders
6. Cosmetics
7. Treated fabrics, papers, adhesives, and bandages

Prevention

Allergic patients should avoid antibacterial (deodorant) soaps and cleansers and underarm deodorants unless such agents are labeled with a complete ingredient list to check for dichlorophen. Patients should be instructed to beware of products listed with only "active agents" or "active ingredients" instead of "ingredients." Dermatologists can assist with choosing a safe soap and antiperspirant. The labels of all cosmetic and personal care products should be carefully read for this agent. Although it is unlikely, such individuals may also react to the following related phenolic antibacterials:

Bithionol (thiobis-dichlorophenol)
Bromochlorosalicylanilide (BCSA) (Multifungin)
Buclosamide (Jadit)
Chloro-2-phenolphenol (Dowacide 32)
Dibromosalicylanilide (DBS) (Dibromsalan)
Fenticlor (thiobis-chlorophenol)
Hexachlorophene (pHisohex)
Tetrachlorosalicylanilide (TCSA)
Trichlorocarbanilide (TCC) (triclocarban)
Triclosan (Irgasan)

Allergic patients should be instructed to be particularly careful to read the labels of cleansers in their workplace. If they are involved in industries related to the production of paper or fabrics, they should be aware that dichlorophen may be used protect such products from mildew.

May be duplicated for use in clinical practice. From Marks JG Jr, Elsner P, DeLeo VA: *Contact and occupational dermatology,* ed 3, St Louis, 2002, Mosby.

have been found to produce the fewest false-positives while still identifying sensitized individuals. Individuals with positive photo–patch test reactions should be questioned extensively to prove clinical relevance.

> **Promethazine and chloropromazine frequently produce photoirritant or false-positive photo–patch test results.**

CHLORPROMAZINE HYDROCHLORIDE

Definition

Chlorpromazine is a phenothiazine that is used as a tranquilizer, sedative, and antiemetic. Chlorpromazine hydrochloride is tested at 0.1% concentration in petrolatum. It produced 1.7% positive photo–patch test reactions in the Scandinavian photopatch test study, 9% (only 11 tested) in the New York group, and 18% in the Mayo Clinic study (1% concentration).

Clinical Aspects

Chlorpromazine and chlorpromazine hydrochloride (Thorazine) are widely used as tranquilizers, antiemetics, and sedatives. Chlorpromazine is used orally and by injection and rectal suppository. It is a well-known photosensitizer when used systemically and produces a classic phototoxic drug reaction with "exaggerated sunburn" and hyperpigmentation.

> **Although chlorpromazine is a common systemic photosensitizer, it infrequently produces photoallergic contact dermatitis, usually in health care workers.**

PACD has been reported much less frequently, primarily in health care workers and individuals involved in the industrial production of the drug. Family members who administer the drug at home to patients have also been involved.

In photo–patch test series, relatively large numbers of patients have positive photo–patch test reactions. For instance, 18% of all individuals tested at the Mayo Clinic had positive photo–patch test results. *None* of those were clinically relevant, however. That series was conducted using the antigen at 1% concentration. Using the 0.1% concentration results in fewer positive results. Even at the lower concentration, 1.7% of patients tested in Scandinavia had positive reactions, most of which were also clinically irrelevant.

Individuals who are exposed and sensitized topically may react not only on the hand but also on the arms, face, and eyelids. "Seborrheic-like" reaction patterns are reported. Cross-reactivity between chlorpromazine and promethazine occur. In addition, chlorpromazine has been reported to cause an immediate urticarial photocontact reaction. Systemic administration could produce systemic photocontact dermatitis in sensitized individuals.

| EXPOSURE LIST | CHLORPROMAZINE HYDROCHLORIDE |

Synonyms and Other Names

Chlorderazin
Chlorpromados
Chlorpromazine
Contonim
Esmind
Fenactil

Novomazina
Promactil
Promazil
Prozil
Thorazine
Wintermin

Uses

Chlorpromazine is used as a tranquilizer in pills, injections, and suppositories.

Prevention

Patients who are allergic to a medication that is used as a tranquilizer or sedative or to prevent vomiting must avoid skin and systemic contact with the agents previously listed. They should be instructed to wear gloves and other protective clothing if they must come into contact with this agent. Such individuals should be told to warn their health care providers that they are allergic to phenothiazines, since they may react to systemic administration of this drug and related agents.

PROMETHAZINE

Definition

Promethazine (Phenergan) is a phenothiazine that is used as an antiemetic and an antihistamine. It is tested at a concentration of 1% in petrolatum. Testing with this antigen produced positive photo–patch test reactions in 45% of patients tested in New York and 1.9% of those tested in the Scandinavian series. At the Mayo Clinic 12% of patients were found to have positive reactions to this antigen at 2% concentration.

Clinical Aspects

Promethazine and promethazine hydrochloride are phenothiazines that are used extensively as antiemetics and less frequently for their antihistaminic properties. They are administered in tablet, liquid, and suppository forms, as well as by injection. They are combined with codeine in cough syrups.

The largest number of reports of photosensitization to promethazine occurred when it was used topically as an antipruritic in Phenergan cream in France in the 1950s. Such a product was never marketed in the United States. Systemic administration does not appear to result in phototoxic drug reactions (as does chlorpromazine), although patients previously sensitized by topical exposure may have a reaction on systemic challenge.

Health care workers are at risk for topical exposure and photosensitization. Cross-reactivity with chlorpromazine frequently occurs. A contact urticaria (plain, not light-induced) with a systemic response to this agent has been reported during patch testing.

EXPOSURE LIST ▷ **PROMETHAZINE**

Synonyms and Other Names

Atosil   Prothazine
Dimapp   Provigan
Fargan   Remsed
Fenazil   Vallgerine
Genphen
Phencen
Phenergan
Promethazine hydrochloride
Prorex

Uses
Promethazine is used as a pill, a syrup, an injection, or a suppository to prevent nausea and vomiting, and as a cough syrup. It may be used in a cream to relieve itch in products manufactured abroad.

Prevention
Patients should be instructed to inform all their health care workers that they are allergic to promethazine and may react to all phenothiazines. Such patients should avoid itch creams that are marketed abroad.

May be duplicated for use in clinical practice. From Marks JG Jr, Elsner P, DeLeo VA: *Contact and occupational dermatology*, ed 3, St Louis, 2002, Mosby.

Photo-patch testing with this antigen frequently produces false-positive responses. Of 11 photosensitive patients tested with this antigen in New York, five (45%) had positive responses; none of these were clinically relevant. A similar lack of relevance was noted in the Scandinavian and Mayo Clinic series. A positive photo-patch test reaction to this antigen requires extensive questioning to reveal its relevance.

Miscellaneous

THIOUREA

Definition

Thiourea (thiocarbamide) is a fixative that is used in photography and photocopy paper as well as an antioxidant in the manufacture of rubber, especially neoprene. It is tested at a concentration of 0.1% in petrolatum. Thiourea was responsible for two (0.1%) positive photo-patch test reactions in 1993 photosensitive patients who were tested in Scandinavia.

Clinical Aspects

Thiourea is an antioxidant that is used as a fixing agent in photography. It is used to remove stains from negatives and to prevent yellowing of copy paper in the diazo or dyeline copying process. It has rarely been reported to cause photosensitization. Patients who are exposed to the copy paper have been reported to have a photosensitivity of the hands, including involvement of the palms. Persistent photosensitivity after discontinuation of antigen contact occurred in reported individuals. If photosensitivity to copy paper is suspected, photo–patch testing with the paper itself should be done.

Plain contact dermatitis to the thiourea in copy paper has also been reported. Alkylthioureas are also used as rubber accelerators. The most common include dimethyl, diethyl, ethylene, dibutyl, and ethylbutyl thioureas. These agents are infrequently used in the manufacture of rubber as compared with the accelerators tested in the standard tray. Rubber containing thioureas has caused plain contact dermatitis when used in insoles, adhesives and adhesive tape, wet suits, and neoprene weather strips. Thioureas are also used in detergents, plastics, textiles, and anticorrosive solutions. None of these other exposures routes, however, has involved photocontact dermatitis.

Concentrations of thiourea as high as 5% have been reported for patch testing, and some reports suggest testing in an aqueous solution instead of a petrolatum vehicle.

Thiourea in photocopy paper may induce photoallergic contact dermatitis. Thioureas in rubber products and adhesives have been reported to cause plain contact dermatitis but not photodermatitis.

BIBLIOGRAPHY

Cronin E: *Contact dermatitis,* London, 1980, Churchill Livingstone.

DeLeo VA, Encarnacion L, Belsito D et al: North American Contact Dermatitis Group photo–patch results: 1992 to 1998, *Am J Contact Dermat,* 10(2):108, 1999.

DeLeo VA, Harber LC: Contact photodermatitis. In Fisher AA, editor: *Contact dermatitis,* ed 3, Philadelphia, 1986, Lea & Febiger.

DeLeo VA, Suarez SM, Maso MJ: Photoallergic contact dermatitis: results of photopatch testing in New York—1985 to 1990, *Arch Dermatol* 128:1513-1518, 1992.

Dromgoole SH, Maibach HI: Contact sensitization and photocontact sensitization of sunscreening agents, *J Am Acad Dermatol* 22:1068-1078, 1990.

Emmett EA: Phototoxicity and photosensitivity reactions. In Adams RM, editor: *Occupational skin disease,* ed 2, Philadelphia, 1990, WB Saunders.

English JSC, White IR, Cronin E: Sensitivity to sunscreens, *Contact Dermatitis* 17:159-162, 1987.

Fisher AA: *Contact dermatitis,* ed 3, Philadelphia, 1986, Lea & Febiger.

Ilarda I, DeLeo VA: Photocontact dermatitis to methyl anthramilate, In preparation, 2001.

Le Coz CJ, Bottlaender A, Scrivener JN et al: Photocontact dermatitis from ketoprofen and tiaprofenic acid: cross-reactivity study in 12 consecutive patients, *Contact Dermatitis,* 38(5):245-252, 1998.

Menz MB, Sigfrid AM, Connolly SM: Photopatch testing: a six-year experience, *J Am Acad Dermatol* 18:1044-1047, 1988.

Nater JP, DeGroot AC: *Unwanted effects of cosmetics and drugs used in dermatology,* ed 2, London, 1985, Elsevier.

Thune P: Contact and photocontact allergy to sunscreens, *Photodermatology* 1:5-9, 1984.

Thune P, Jansen C, Wennersten G et al: The Scandinavian multicenter photopatch study: 1980 to 1985—final report, *Photodermatology* 5:261-269, 1988.

Trevisi CV, Chieregatolg, Tosti A: Sunscreen sensitization: a three-year study, *Dermatology* 189:55-57, 1994.

Von der Leun TC, Dekreek EJ, Deensta-van Leeuwen M et al: Photosensitivity owing to thiourea, *Arch Dermatol* 113:1611, 1977.

CHAPTER 10

Plants

The thousands of plant species and their numerous chemical products make the study of phytodermatitis daunting. The purpose of this chapter is not to review the entire subject but to discuss in some detail the most important plants that cause allergic contact dermatitis. The vernacular names will be used to identify these plants, since they are the ones most commonly recognized by the investigating clinician and the patient. Scientific names are included under the synonyms. Irritant plants are not discussed because in most cases the irritant nature of the plant is already known by the patient. Allergic contact dermatitis to plants, on the other hand, is often unrecognized by the patient and requires astute investigative skills by the clinician. For less common causes of phytodermatitis, the reader is referred to the following textbooks dealing with this subject:

1. *Plant Contact Dermatitis* by Benezra, Ducombs, Sell, and Foussereau, Toronto, 1985, BC Decker.
2. *Botanical Dermatology* by Mitchell and Rook, Vancouver, Canada, 1979, Greengrass.
3. *Woods Injurious to Human Health* by Hausen, Berlin, 1981, Walter de Gruyter.
4. *Plants and the Skin* by Lovell, Oxford, 1993, Blackwell.

Signs of Plant Dermatitis

Suspect plant dermatitis if the person has the following:
1. Summer flare
2. Exposed skin affected
3. Hand and/or facial dermatitis
4. Occupational or hobby-related exposure to plants

Investigating Plant Dermatitis

The investigation of contact dermatitis from plants is complicated by the huge number of plant species and multitude of plant products that they produce. There are over half a million known plant species and over 11,000 naturally occurring compounds from plants. Further complicating the matter is the fact that a particular chemical or product within the plant may vary depending on the genetic constitution of the plant, the anatomic portion of the plant sample, the age of the plant, and environmental factors such as climate, moisture, and soil. The commercial availability of plant antigens is limited, which forces the inquisitive physician to patch test with portions of the plant or to make plant extracts with the help of a pharmacist or biochemist.

The first step in investigating contact dermatitis from plants begins with recognizing this as a possibility. Sometimes this is quite easy in the case of a florist, gardener, or forester. The episodic nature of the dermatitis and the association with the workplace makes one suspect plants as a likely cause of contact dermatitis in these individuals (Box 10-1). For the housewife who has indoor plants such as *Primula obconica,* the etiologic factors may be more obscure. How often do we ask the housewife with hand or facial dermatitis what plants she cares for at home? In either setting, as a hobby or as an occupation, the number of plants the patient may come in contact with can be numerous. To illustrate this point, we reported a woman who had recurrent allergic contact dermatitis of the hands each summer for 3 years. Typically the dermatitis was most severe during the months when she was gardening outdoors. Patch tests to 14 plants from her garden revealed positive reactions to portions of nasturtium *(Tropaeolum majus).* Results of further testing with an acetone extract of the plant and the isothiocyanate allergens were positive and confirmed allergic contact dermatitis from this popular flowering annual plant. Her dermatitis completely cleared when she avoided nasturtiums.

Once it is recognized that plant contact dermatitis may be occurring, the clinical investigation begins (Box 10-2). The patient should bring in all suspected plants including weeds with which there has been contact. An attempt to identify the plants should be made before patch testing so that known irritant plants can be avoided. Positive patch test responses to irritant plants are, of course, expected. Most of the time the plant is referred to by its common name. This is not precise nomenclature. The botanical identification and proper names are derived from the *International Code of Botanical Nomenclature.* The help of a botanist, preferably a plant taxonomist, who may be found at a university botany department, a botanic garden, or a state or federal department of agriculture, may be required. The first classification that had widespread acceptance was conceived by Linnaeus in 1753. He assembled plants into groups on the basis of a floral morphologic similarity that was published in *Systema Naturae*. Subsequently, recent classifications have considered the biochemistry, anatomy, genetics, and cytology of the plants. For example, Linnaeus placed poison ivy in the genus *Rhus*. More recently, it was put in the restricted genus *Toxicodendron* because of a number of characteristics that separate poison ivy from *Rhus* species.

If there is a limited supply of the plant material, the plants should be divided into three parts as recommended by Mitchell and Rook (1979). These parts are used for patch testing, for botanic identification, and for making plant extracts. Storing plant materials is best done by freezing rather than air drying, which may significantly alter the plant chemicals responsible for the dermatitis. Patch testing is done with the actual plants with which the patient comes in contact, as well as botanically related species if indicated. Portions of the plant, leaf, stem, and petal are gently crushed and applied under tape in the usual manner for patch testing. For plants of unknown irritancy, control patch tests on 10 to 20 normal subjects are essential for interpreting patch test results. Patch testing bulbs is accomplished with the moist, fleshy, outer layers of the bulb underneath the thin, dried outer scale. To rule out allergic contact dermatitis to woods, patch testing with sawdust mixed 10% by weight in petrolatum is usually reliable. For some plants the specific allergenic chemical or extract is available for patch testing to confirm an allergy. The risk of sensitization by testing to plant allergens or portions of plants is well known. For example, poison ivy is not usually patch tested because it has a significant sensitizing capacity. High concentrations of wood extracts, urushiol from poison ivy or poison oak, primin from primrose, and alantolactone from mums and other Compositae plants have actively sensitized individuals by patch testing. Photo–patch testing can also be accomplished with plant materials (see Chapter 9). It should be pointed out, however, that photo–patch testing plants containing psoralens is useless, since a phototoxic reaction can be expected.

Different types of cutaneous reactions to plants have been described. These include allergic contact dermatitis, irritant contact dermatitis, photodermatitis, and contact urticaria. Selected plants causing these reactions and the putative

Table 10-1 — Plants Causing Allergic Contact Dermatitis

Common Name	Botanic Name	Allergen
Wild feverfew	*Parthenium hysterophorus*	Sesquiterpene lactones: parthenin, hymenin
Lichen	*Primelia, Evernia, Cladonia,* and *Usnea* species	Usnic acid, atranorin, evernic acid
Liverwort	*Frullania* species	Sesquiterpene lactones: frullanolide
Mum	*Chrysanthemum indicum* and *C. morifolium*	Sesquiterpene lactones: alantolactone, parthenolide, arteglasin A
Peruvian lily	*Alstroemeria* species	Tuliposide A
Pine tree	*Pinus* species	Colophony (rosin)
Poison ivy	*Toxicodendron radicans* and *T. rydbergii*	Urushiol: pentadecylcatechols
Poison oak	*Toxicodendron diversilobum* and *T. toxicarium*	Urushiol: heptadecylcatechols
Primrose	*Primula obconica*	Primin
Ragweed	*Ambrosia* species	Sesquiterpene lactones: frullanolide
Tulip	*Tulipa* species	Tuliposide A
Honduras balsam	*Toluifera pereirae*	Balsam of Peru

Table 10-2 — Plants Causing Irritant Contact Dermatitis*

Common Name	Botanic Name	Irritant
Black mustard	*Brassica nigra*	Isothiocyanates
Buttercup	*Ranunculus bulbosus*	Protoanemonin
Croton	*Croton tiglium*	Phorbol esters
Dumbcane	*Dieffenbachia* species	Calcium oxalate
Manchineel tree	*Hippomane mancinella*	Phorbol esters
May apple	*Podophyllum peltatum*	Podophyllin resin
Pencil tree	*Euphorbia tirucalli*	Triterpene alcohols
Prickly pear	*Opuntia* species	Spines

*Small sampling of the many plants that are irritating, mainly from the families Ranunculaceae, Cruciferae, Euphorbiaeae, and Capparidaceae.

agent are summarized in Tables 10-1 to 10-4. Allergic contact dermatitis, potentially the most troublesome and obscure cause of cutaneous reactions, is discussed in more detail in this chapter. Certain types of plants tend to elicit a characteristic eruption. Weeds tend to cause a chronic lichenified dermatitis in the exposed skin of the face, neck, and arms that simulates photodermatitis. Ragweed is an ex-

Table 10-3 — Plants Causing Photodermatitis*

Common Name	Botanic Name	Comment
Bergamot	*Citrus bergamia*	Berloque dermatitis
Celery	*Apium graveolens*	Fungal infection accentuates
Common rue	*Ruta graveolens*	Insect repellant
Gas plant	*Dictamnus albus*	
Lime	*Citrus aurantifolia*	Drinks
Mokihana	*Pelea anisata*	Hawaiian leis
Parsnip	*Pastinaca sativa*	

The photosensitizers are furocomarins that include psoralens.
*Selected plants from the families Umbelliferae and Rutaceae.

Table 10-4 — Plants Causing Contact Urticaria

Common Name	Botanic Name	Urticant
Chili pepper	*Capsicum* species	Capsaicin
Cowhage	*Mucuna pruriens*	Itch powder: mucanain
Endive	*Chichorium endivia*	?
Great nettle	*Urtica dioica*	Stinging hairs containing histamine, acetylcholine, 5-hydroxytryptamine

ample of this type of airborne phytodermatitis. Flowers and bulbs generally cause a dry, scaling, fissured dermatitis of the hands, particularly the fingertips. Streaky, linear, blotchy, asymmetric, acute and subacute dermatitis is typical for poison ivy and poison oak. Sawdust dermatitis affects the eyelids, face, neck, and skin folds such as the genital area, where the dust settles. A phytodermatitis is usually seasonal, with the exception of the year-round exposure that florists and housewives may experience.

BIBLIOGRAPHY

Beaman JH: Plant taxonomy, *Clin Dermatol* 4:23-30, 1986.
Benezra C, Ducombs G, Sell Y et al: *Plant contact dermatitis,* Toronto, 1985, BC Decker.
Bowers AG: Phytophotodermatitis, *Am J Contact Dermat* 10:89-93, 1999.
Diamond SP, Wiener SG, Marks JG: Allergic contact dermatitis to nasturtium, *Dermatol Clin* 8:77-80, 1990.
Epstein WL: Irritant contact dermatitis: house and garden plants, *J Toxicol–Cut Ocular Toxicol* 19 (4):207-235, 2000.
Epstein WL: House and garden plants. In Jackson EM, Goldner R, editors, *Irritant contact dermatitis,* New York, 1990, Marcel Dekker.
Guin JD: Patch testing to plants: some practical aspects of what has become an esoteric area of contact dermatitis, *Am J Contact Dermat* 6:232-235, 1995.
Lovell CR: *Plants and the skin,* Oxford, 1993, Blackwell.

McGovern TW: The language of plants, *Am J Contact Dermat* 10:45-47, 1999.

Mitchell J, Rook A: Diagnosis of contact dermatitis from plants, *Int J Dermatol* 16:257-264, 1977.

Mitchell J, Rook A: *Botanical dermatology: plants and plant products injurious to the skin,* Vancouver, Canada, 1979, Greengrass.

Norton SA: Botanical heritage of dermatology. In Avalos J, Maibach HI, editors: *Dermatologic botany,* Boca Raton, Fla, 2000, CRC Press.

Schmidt RJ: Plants. In Adams RM, editor: *Occupational skin disease,* ed 2, Philadelphia, 1990, WB Saunders.

Stoner JG, Rasmussen JE: Plant dermatitis, *J Am Acad Dermatol* 9:1-15, 1983.

Zug KA, Marks JG: Occupational dermatitis from plants and woods. In Adams RM, editor: *Occupational skin disease,* ed 3, Philadelphia, 1999, WB Saunders.

Specific Plants

ALSTROEMERIA SPECIES

Definition

The genus *Alstroemeria* is a popular cut flower because of its beautiful, trumpet-shaped, lilylike flowers (Plate 66A). Patch tests can be done with portions of the *Alstroemeria* plant (Plate 66B) and its principal allergens tuliposide A (0.1%) or α-methylene-γ-butyrolactone (0.01%) in petrolatum.

> The genus *Alstroemeria* is the most common cause of allergic contact dermatitis affecting florists.

Clinical Aspects

The genus *Alstroemeria* is native to Central and South America and grows in the desert and mountains. In the early 1960s the Dutch began breeding projects to develop varieties of *Alstroemeria* for year-round cut flowers. Since then, this showy flower has become quite popular in Europe and subsequently in the United States. Its natural beauty, numerous varieties, year-round availability, and long-lasting flower have made it popular with florists. There are over 50 species of *Alstroemeria,* of which *A. aurantiaca Don* and *A. ligtu L* are the most popular with growers in Holland, South America, and California. The flower resembles the lily with inner petals that are always bicolored and streaked or dappled. A number of colors are available including red, pink, yellow, purple, white, salmon, and apricot.

Allergic contact dermatitis from the genus *Alstroemeria* was originally reported from Europe and subsequently recognized in the United States. It typically affects floral workers, specifically designers and arrangers, who develop chronic, fissured, dermatitis of the fingers from prolonged, repeated contact with the cut flowers. The fingertips are typically tender, erythematous, fissured, and hyperkeratotic and mimic the clinical appearance of "tulip fingers," a type of allergic contact dermatitis in tulip workers. Some floral workers may also have spread of the dermatitis to the hands, forearms, and face. In addition to chronic dermatitis, depigmentation at patch test and dermatitic sites has been reported.

Individuals who are sensitized by tulip bulbs are generally allergic to *Alstroemeria* species and vice versa because the two plants share the common allergen

Synonyms and Other Names
Inca lily
Peruvian lily

Uses
The *Alstroemeria* genus is a popular cut flower that is used by florists in table arrangements and bouquets. It has a distinctive, attractive, lilylike flower set on a slender, leafy stem.

Prevention
Allergic contact dermatitis due to *Alstroemeria* species affects florists and floriculture workers who have repeated and prolonged contact with this flower. It is unlikely that an occasional casual contact with *Alstroemeria* would cause sensitization. Prevention of contact dermatitis may require banishing this flower from the workplace. Nitrile latex gloves are protective.

May be duplicated for use in clinical practice. From Marks JG Jr, Elsner P, DeLeo VA: *Contact and occupational dermatology,* ed 3, St Louis, 2002, Mosby.

tuliposide A. Although the amount of tuliposide A is not uniform within floral species or within portions of a single plant, patch testing with the petal, stem, and leaf generally gives positive reactions. Tuliposide A is a precursor of the sensitizing component tulipalin A, α-methylene-γ-butyrolactone, which results from the hydrolysis of tuliposide A and lactonization of its aglycone.

> The allergens in *Alstroemeria* species are *tuliposide A* and α-methylene-γ-butyrolactone. Patch testing can be done with α-methylene-γ-butyrolactone, which is available commercially, or with the petal, stem, or leaf from the plant.

BIBLIOGRAPHY

Adams RM, Daily AD, Brancaccio RR et al: *Alstroemeria:* a new and potent allergen for florists, *Dermatol Clin* 8:73-76, 1990.

Bjorkner BE: Contact allergy and depigmentation from *Alstroemeria, Contact Dermatitis* 8:178-184, 1982.

Christensen LP: Direct release of the allergen tulipalin A from *Alstroemeria* cut flowers: a possible source of airborne contact dermatitis? *Contact Dermatitis* 41:320-324, 1999.

Christensen LP, Kristiansen K: A simple HPLC method for the isolation and quantification of the allergens tuliposide A and tulipalin A in *Alstroemeria, Contact Dermatitis* 32:199-203, 1995.

Hausen BM, Prater E, Schubert H: The sensitizing capacity of *Alstroemeria* cultivars in man and guinea pig, *Contact Dermatitis* 9:46-54, 1983.

Marks JG: Allergic contact dermatitis to *Alstroemeria, Arch Dermatol* 124:914-915, 1988.

McGovern TW: *Alstroemeria L.* (Peruvian lily), *Am J Contact Dermat* 10:172-176, 1999.

Rook A: Dermatitis from *Alstroemeria:* altered clinical pattern and probable increasing incidence of contact dermatitis to *Alstroemeria, Contact Dermatitis* 7:355-356, 1981.

Rycroft RJG, Calnan CD: *Alstroemeria* dermatitis, *Contact Dermatitis* 7:284, 1981.

Santucci B, Picardo M, Iavarone C et al: Contact dermatitis to *Alstroemeria, Contact Dermatitis* 12:215-219, 1985.

Thiboutot DM, Hamory BH, Marks JG: Dermatoses among floral shop workers, *J Am Acad Dermatol* 22:54-58, 1990.

Van Ketel WG, Verspyck AW, Neering H: Contact eczema from *Alstroemeria, Contact Dermatitis* 1:323-324, 1975.

CHRYSANTHEMUM

Definition

The chrysanthemums used by florists comprise over 500 varieties (cultivars) generally referred to as *Chrysanthemum indicum* or *Chrysanthemum morifolium*, with the latter more recently reclassified as *Dendranthema grandiflora*. These beautifully flowering plants are commonly referred to as mums and are one of the causes of allergic contact dermatitis in florists. Patch testing is best accomplished with the stem, leaf, and flower petal of the individual plant to which the patient has been exposed. The results of patch testing with the sesquiterpene lactone mix or specific sesquiterpene lactones such as alantolactone or arteglasin A is often, but not uniformly, positive in patients with chrysanthemum dermatitis.

Clinical Aspects

Chrysanthemums are a favorite cut flower and are found in most floral arrangements. Their hardiness and great variety of colored and shaped flowers make mums a staple. Chrysanthemums, particularly autumn-flowering chrysanthemums, are also a popular garden flower. Chrysanthemums belong to the family Compositae (also known as Asteraceae), which is one of the largest plant families and contains approximately 20,000 species. They are found in most regions of the world and are generally herbaceous plants (Table 10-5). A large number of Compositae members are weeds, in addition to those that are ornamental. Just a few are cultivated as vegetables. The Compositae family has gained dermatologic interest, since members of this family cause a significant amount of contact dermatitis. Besides chrysanthemums, ragweed (*Ambrosia* species) and feverfew (*Parthenium* species) are discussed in this chapter.

> **Sesquiterpene lactones are the allergens in chrysanthemums and other Compositae plants (e.g., ragweed and feverfew).**

The allergens in the Compositae family are sesquiterpene lactones. These terpenoid plant constituents have a number of significant biologic effects including antitumor, cytotoxic, antibacterial, and antifungal activity. Over 3,000 sesquiterpene lactones have been isolated and identified, with some being synthesized. Sesquiterpene lactones have been found not only in plants of the Compositae family but also in other unrelated plants, importantly in liverworts (*Frullania* species). The sesquiterpene lactones are produced in glandular trichomes (hairlike structures) on the plant surface. It is from contact with these trichomes that dermatitis develops. Several sesquiterpene lactones have been isolated for patch testing, but testing is complicated by the following important variables: (1) the amount

Table 10-5	Most Familiar of Over 20,000 Species of Compositae	
Artichoke	Indian plantain
Aster	Ironweed
Black-eyed Susan	Joe-pye weed
Boneset	Lettuce
Broomweed	Marigold
Burdock	Pearly everlasting
Butterweed	Pyrethrum
Chamomile	Rabbit tobacco
Chicory	Ragweed
Chrysanthemum	Ragwort
Cocklebur	Sagebrush
Coreopsis	Sneezeweed
Cornflower	Stinkweed
Cosmos	Stoksia
Costus	Sunflower
Daisy	Tansy
Dahlia	Tarragon
Dandelion	Thistle
Dusty miller	Tickweed
Endive	White snakeroot
Feverfew	Wormwood
Fleabane	Yarrow
Giallardia	Zinnia
Goldenrod	

Modified from Crounse RJ: *J Am Acad Dermatol* 2:417-424, 1980.

and type of sesquiterpene lactones can vary among different cultivars of the same species and (2) no single sesquiterpene lactone is sufficient to screen for sensitivity to chrysanthemums. Thus the actual chrysanthemum plant to which the patient has been exposed must be tested. In a given patient cross-reactivity cannot be predicted reliably. Some cultivars elicit dermatitis, others do not. Over 100 of the identified sesquiterpene lactones are potentially allergic. A prerequisite structural configuration of these allergic sesquiterpenes is the presence of an exocyclic α-methylene group attached to a γ-lactone ring. These sesquiterpenes lactones are usually lipophilic and unsubstituted at C6 or C8. If the α-methylene group is reduced, allergenicity is lost.

The clinical picture of allergic contact dermatitis due to chrysanthemums and the other Compositae is quite similar. Sesquiterpene lactone–induced dermatitis can be acute dermatitis, but more commonly it is a chronic, diffuse, erythematous, lichenified eruption of the exposed skin that resembles photodermatitis. Involvement of the upper eyelids and the retroauricular and submental regions of the head and neck helps to differentiate Compositae dermatitis from photodermatitis. Although not definitively proved, the most likely mechanism of this diffuse dermatitis is from airborne exposure to the plant trichomes containing the allergen. Often the fingers or hands are the initial site of involvement among florists

| EXPOSURE LIST | *FRULLANIA* (Liverworts) |

Synonyms and Other Names
Frullania species

Uses
Liverworts have no commercial value.

Prevention
Liverworts are primitive mosslike plants that are found on the bark of trees and on rocks in humid areas of the forest. They have caused dermatitis involving the exposed skin of the hands, arms, neck, and head that is referred to as "cedar wood poisoning" and "woodcutter's eczema."

Forest workers who have contact with the bark of trees, such as "fallers," who fell trees, are most often affected. In most cases, giving up work in the forest and changing jobs to occupations where there is no exposure to liverworts is required. Patients who are allergic to liverworts may also have an allergy to members of the Compositae family of plants, including chrysanthemums, tansy, and ragweed.

May be duplicated for use in clinical practice. From Marks JG Jr, Elsner P, DeLeo VA: *Contact and occupational dermatology,* ed 3, St Louis, 2002, Mosby.

sesquiterpene lactone mix at 0.1% concentration in petrolatum, however, is a good screening allergen for *Frullania* sensitivity.

> *Frullania* species (liverworts) are members of the Jubulaceae family of plants. They have sesquiterpene lactone allergens like plants in the family Compositae. The sesquiterpene lactone mix is a good screening allergen.

Clinical Aspects

Frullania are small, reddish brown plants that are found in the humid forests of the Pacific Northwest, France, and other regions of Europe. Allergic contact dermatitis from *Frullania* resembles the dermatitis caused by Compositae plants that have similar sesquiterpene lactone allergens. It is a chronic, erythematous, lichenified dermatitis affecting exposed skin in a photodermatitis-like appearance. The main sesquiterpene lactone found in *Frullania* species is frullanolide, but patients also react to alantolactone.

> *Frullania* produces a chronic allergic contact dermatitis in foresters that mimics photodermatitis.

BIBLIOGRAPHY

Julian CG, Bowers PW, Paton JA: *Frullania* dermatitis, *Contact Dermatitis* 43:119-121, 2000.
Mitchell JC: Industrial aspects of 112 cases of allergic contact dermatitis from *Frullania* in British Columbia during a 10-year period, *Contact Dermatitis* 7:268-269, 1981.
Mitchell JC: *Frullania* (liverwort) phytodermatitis (woodcutter's eczema), *Clin Dermatol* 4:62-64, 1986.
Quirce S, Tabar AI, Muro MD, Olaguibel JM: Airborne contact dermatitis from *Frullania, Contact Dermatitis* 30:73-76, 1994.

GREVILLEA SPECIES

There are dozens of species of *Grevillea* in Queensland, Australia, although only two have been implicated as responsible for allergic contact dermatitis. These plants have been imported to other regions of the world. *Grevillea banksii* (Bank's grevillea) is a tall shrub or slender, small tree that produces Kahili flowers, which only have been used in Hawaii to make garlands (leis) and bouquets. This flower has been responsible for the allergic contact dermatitis of women who wear them. *Grevillea robusta* (silk oak) is a graceful, fern-leaved plant that is used for landscaping and as a source of wood for barrels and furniture. Acute allergic contact dermatitis to *G. robusta* has been reported among powerline workers in Los Angeles and among those who have contact with its sawdust. The allergic component of *G. robusta* is grevillol, a resorcinol. No cross-reactivity occurs between *G. robusta* and *G. banksii*.

BIBLIOGRAPHY

Arnold HL: Dermatitis due to the blossom of *Grevillea banksii, Arch Dermatol Syph* 45:1037-1051, 1942.

Lampe KF: Dermatitis-producing plants of South Florida and Hawaii, *Clin Dermatol* 4:83-86, 1986.

May SB: Dermatitis due to *Grevillea robusta* (Australian silk oak), *Arch Dermatol* 82:1006, 1962.

LICHENS

> **Allergic contact dermatitis to lichens from usnic acid, atranorin, and so forth occurs in forestry workers, gardeners, and individuals using perfumed products.**

Lichens are composed of algae and fungi that live in symbiosis. There are thousands of species of lichens, and they are found worldwide on rocks, trees, concrete, and bricks. Allergic contact dermatitis from these plants usually affects forest workers and woodcutters and simulates a photosensitive eruption similar to that seen with *Frullania* species and with Compositae plants such as ragweed.

> **The lichen extracts oak moss and tree moss cause fragrance allergy from aftershave lotions.**

Lichen extracts, particularly oak moss and tree moss, are fragrances commonly added to aftershaves because of their "masculine" scent (see Chapter 7). The allergens in lichens include usnic acid, atranorin, evernic acid, fumarprotocetraric acid, and other lichen acids. Forest workers who are allergic to lichen acids often have concomitant sensitivity to the sesquiterpene lactones found in liverworts (*Frullania* species). This, however, is not a true cross-reaction between lichen acids and sesquiterpene lactones, but rather cosensitivity.

BIBLIOGRAPHY

Dahlquist I, Fregert S: Contact allergy to atranorin in lichens and perfumes, *Contact Dermatitis* 6:111-119, 1980.

Hahn M, Lischka G, Pfeifle J, Wirth V: A case of contact dermatitis from lichens in Southern Germany, *Contact Dermatitis* 32:55-56, 1995.

Quirino AP, Barros MA: Occupational contact dermatitis from lichens and *Frullania, Contact Dermatitis* 33:68, 1995.

Rafanelli S, Bacchilega R, Stanganelli I, Rafanelli A: Contact dermatitis from usnic acid in vaginal ovules, *Contact Dermatitis* 33:271-272, 1995.

Stinchi C, Guerrini V, Ghetti E et al: Contact dermatitis from lichens, *Contact Dermatitis* 36:309-310, 1997.

Thune P, Solberg Y, McFadden N et al: Perfume allergy due to oak moss and other lichens, *Contact Dermatitis* 8:396-400, 1982.

POISON IVY AND POISON OAK

Definition

Poison ivy and poison oak (Plates 67 and 68) are members of the Anacardiaceae family of plants (Table 10-6) and belong in the genus *Toxicodendron*. There are two species of poison ivy, *T. radicans* and *T. rydbergii. T. radicans* is a climbing vine that is found in the eastern United States, and *T. rydbergii* is a nonclimbing dwarf shrub found in the northern and western United States. Poison oak also has two species: the eastern *T. toxicarium* and the western *T. diversilobum*. Patch testing to portions of the plant or its sap, urushiol, is usually not done in the United States because of the potential of actively sensitizing the patient. However, in Japan a low concentration of urushiol, in petrolatum, is routinely used for patch testing. At least 50% of the adult population in North America is allergic to poison ivy or poison oak.

Table 10-6	Anacardiaceae Family
Toxicodendron Genus	
Poison ivy	
T. radicans (climbing)	
T. rydbergii (nonclimbing)	
Poison oak	
T. diversilobum (western United States)	
T. toxicarium (eastern United States)	
Poison sumac	
T. vernix	
Other Members	
Cashew: *Anacardium occidentale*	
Indian marking nut: *Semecarpus anacardium*	
Japanese lacquer: *Rhus vernicifera*	
Mango: *Mangifera indica*	

Clinical Aspects

Allergic contact dermatitis from poison ivy or oak usually becomes evident as an acute papulovesicular eruption characterized by linear streaks (Plate 52), sharp margins, and geographic outlines (Plate 23). The vesicles often coalesce into bullae. Urticarial or cellulitic-appearing plaques may also occur. Secondary changes include weeping, crusting, edema, and excoriations. Diffuse, confluent, severe dermatitis of the exposed skin of the head, neck, and arms is produced from the smoke of the burning plant. Occasionally, black dots or streaks of dried urushiol surrounded by dermatitis may also be seen. The eruption is accompanied by

> **Poison ivy/oak allergic contact dermatitis typically appears as linear streaks of papulovesicles. The dermatitis may also look urticarial, cellulitic, and have black dots or streaks from dried urushiol.**

marked itching and usually begins within 24 to 48 hours after contact with the plant. It is not infrequent, however, for new areas of dermatitis to develop for several days after the initial outbreak. This has led to the mistaken belief that blister fluid can spread the dermatitis to new regions. Urushiol is absorbed relatively quickly into the skin, thus making it necessary to wash with soap and water within 5 to 10 minutes after exposure to prevent dermatitis. Inanimate objects such as clothing and animal fur may be contaminated with urushiol and cause allergic contact dermatitis in individuals who have no direct contact with the plant. Poison ivy or oak dermatitis usually occurs in the summer, when sensitive individuals have contact with the plant from outdoor activities. Allergic contact dermatitis can also occur in the winter from residual vines on logs used for firewood.

> **The allergens in poison ivy and oak are *catechols,* which are found in the plant's sap, *urushiol.***

The allergens responsible for poison ivy or oak allergic contact dermatitis are contained within the resinous sap material, termed *urushiol.* The quantity and composition of urushiols vary with the genetic composition (genotype) of the plant and the environment in which it grows. Urushiol is composed of a mixture of catechol with a straight alk(en)yl side chain at the C3 position. The different catechols vary in the degree of saturation and length of their side chains. Poison ivy urushiol contains predominantly 3-pentadecylcatechols (C15 side chain), whereas poison oak contains 3-heptadecylcatechols (C17 side chain). Changes in the structure of these compounds alter their antigenicity. Substitution on the catechol ring reduces antigenicity. When the side chain is desaturated and longer, antigenicity is increased. The 3-*n*-catechol haptens are thought to be changed to electrophilic *o*-quinones that react with a carrier protein on the surface of Langerhans' cells and are then presented to sensitized T lymphocytes. If the hapten and carrier protein are linked via a sulfhydryl bond, reduced allergenicity is produced through selective induction of suppressor T cells. Linkage via an amino nucleophile leads to selective induction of T-effector cells and allergic contact dermatitis. Thiol nucleophiles react at the C6 position, whereas amino nucleophiles react at the C5 position. Blockage at the C5 position, for example, with 5-methyl-3-pentadecylcatechol, results in a weak sensitizer and a good tolerogen because pentadecylcatechol metabolism is protected from nucleophilic attack by amino groups.

Poison ivy or oak–sensitive individuals can react to other plants of the Anacardiaceae family (Table 10-6) causing allergic contact dermatitis because they share chemically similar allergens. Within the United States, poison sumac *(Toxicodendron vernix)* is well known. Poison sumac is a small shrub or tree that grows in moist, swampy areas. Its stems bear an odd number of smooth-edged, pointed leaflets. Other members of the Anacardiaceae family that have caused allergic contact dermatitis in poison ivy or oak–sensitive individuals include the cashew nut, mango, Indian marking nut, and Japanese lacquer trees. Perioral dermatitis and cheilitis are well-known consequences of eating unpeeled mangos, which contain the allergen in the fruit's skin. The black pigment from the Indian marking nut is used to identify laundry in India and has caused allergic contact dermatitis in poison ivy or oak–sensitive individuals who had their clothing marked with this resin. Allergic contact dermatitis of the buttocks has been caused by toilet seats varnished with the black sap from the Japanese lacquer tree; also, occupationally induced dermatitis has occurred in workers who coat decorative articles with the raw lacquer. Cheilitis, stomatitis, proctitis, and pruritus have occurred after eating ginkgo fruit pulp.

> **Individuals who are sensitive to poison ivy and oak can also develop allergic contact dermatitis to other plants in the Anacardiaceae family—cashew, mango, lacquer tree, and marking nut.**

Perhaps the most interesting example of cross-sensitivity among members of the Anacardiaceae family has been caused by cashew shell oil. A large epidemic of poison ivy-like dermatitis *(systemic eczematous contact dermatitis)* was reported by Marks and others shortly after the consumption of improperly processed imported cashew nuts contaminated with the oil from their shells. Fifty-four poison ivy–sensitive individuals had a pruritic, erythematous eruption that was accentuated in the flexural areas of the body. Some had blistering of the mouth and rectal itching. Another example of systemic contact dermatitis producing maculopapular, erythema multiforme–like, and erythroderma eruptions occurred in Korea, where lacquer tree folk medicine is ingested to cure gastrointestinal illnesses.

In contrast, another investigation by Reginella and others (1989) revealed hyposensitization to poison ivy after working in a cashew shell oil processing factory that modified and converted the oil into a solid particulate that was used to make brake linings. Those workers who had a preemployment history of poison ivy sensitivity developed an eczematous eruption characteristic of allergic contact dermatitis after beginning work in the facility. The eruption lasted about 3 weeks and then subsided, with the workers having no further dermatitis. Approximately 10% of the new workers did not have clearing of the dermatitis and required a change of employment. The workers who became hardened to cashew shell oil noticed a decreased sensitivity or no sensitivity to poison ivy and oak. Patch testing to urushiol confirmed this history. These results implied that hyposensitization to poison ivy

---

EXPOSURE LIST ▶ **POISON IVY AND POISON OAK**

Synonyms and Other Names

Black mercury vine
Rhus
Three-leaved ivy
Toxicodendron species

T. diversilobum and *T. toxicarium* (poison oak)
T. radicans and *T. rydbergii* (poison ivy)
Trailing or climbing sumac

Uses

Ointments containing poison ivy and oak extracts are available in Europe for treatment of muscle aches.

Prevention

Exposure to poison ivy and oak is usually from outdoor activities such as gardening, hiking, lumbering, and fire fighting. Exposure can also occur from the poison ivy or oak sap being carried on inanimate objects such as clothing and the fur of animals. Furthermore, in the winter, logs used for wood-burning stoves and fireplaces may contain the dried vines of poison ivy. These dried vines can still cause dermatitis. Other members of the Anacardiaceae plant family—poison sumac, mango, cashew, Japanese lacquer tree, and Indian marking nut—can cause allergic contact dermatitis in poison ivy or oak–sensitive individuals.

The best way of preventing allergic contact dermatitis from poison ivy or oak is by recognizing the plant and avoiding it. When this fails, washing with soap and water within 5 to 10 minutes after exposure can prevent the dermatitis. Care should be taken in burning leaves or other brush that contains poison ivy and oak because the smoke contains droplets of the sap that can cause severe dermatitis on the exposed skin of the arms, face, and neck. Rubber gloves usually do not protect the hands against poison ivy. For contaminated clothing, ordinary washing is usually effective in removing the resin. Hyposensitization with extracts of poison ivy and oak has *not* been proven effective scientifically and is not recommended. Inactivating the poison ivy or oak resin by a barrier cream before its absorption into the skin is an attractive alternative. A lotion containing quaternium-18-bentonite (Ivy Block) is very effective in preventing poison ivy and oak dermatitis.

An excellent educational pamphlet entitled "Poison Ivy" is available from the American Academy of Dermatology.* It contains color photographs of poison ivy, oak, and sumac plants and poison ivy dermatitis. Poison ivy recognition, treatment, prevention, and common myths are discussed.

Herbicides are available that kill poison ivy and oak. None of these are specific for these poisonous plants and therefore can destroy surrounding vegetation, depending on the type. A convenient preparation, Ortho Poison Oak and Poison Ivy Killer Formula II (Chevron Chemical Co., San Francisco, CA), contains Triclopyr, a herbicide that kills bushy weeds and woody plants such as poison ivy and oak, willow, oak, grapes, blackberries, and honeysuckle.

May be duplicated for use in clinical practice. From Marks JG Jr, Elsner P, DeLeo VA: *Contact and occupational dermatology,* ed 3, St Louis, 2002, Mosby.
*930 N. Meacham Road, Schaumburg, IL 60173-4965.

---

and oak occurred in those employees after development of hardening to cashew shell oil. Cashew shell oil contains cardol and anacardic acid, which are immunochemically similar to the catechol found in poison ivy and oak. Hyposensitization to urushiol has also been observed in Japanese lacquer workers who coat decorative articles (lacquerware) with raw lacquer from the lacquer tree.

BIBLIOGRAPHY

Brook I, Frazier EH, Yeager JK: Microbiology of infected poison ivy dermatitis, *Br J Dermatol* 142:943-946, 2000.

Epstein WL: The poison ivy picker of Pennypack Park: the continuing saga of poison ivy, *J Invest Dermatol* 88(suppl):7-12, 1987.

dermatitis involving the hands, face, and neck occurs. Characteristically the fingertips are affected as a consequence of picking off the dead flowers and leaves. This can easily be misdiagnosed as dyshidrosis.

Primin, the allergen in *P. obconica* (2-methoxy-6-pentyl-1-4 benzoquinone), is found in tiny hairs (trichomes) on the flower stalk and leaves. The amount of allergen that is produced varies according to the season (the highest amount is present during the spring and summer months) the cultivation method, and the horticultural variety. Primin can be extracted from the plant but is also available commercially as a synthetic chemical. Another potential allergen, miconidin (2-methoxy-6-pentyl-1,4-dihydroxybenzene) has been isolated from *P. obconica.*

> **Patch testing is best done with synthetic *primin,* the allergen in *Primula obconica.***

BIBLIOGRAPHY

Aplin CG, Lovell CR: Hardy *Primula* species and allergic contact dermatitis, *Contact Dermatitis* 42:11, 2000.

Christensen LP, Larsen E: Direct emission of the allergen primin from intact *Primula obconica* plants, *Contact Dermatitis* 42:149-153, 2000.

Dooms-Goossens A, Biesemans G, Vandaele M et al: *Primula* dermatitis: more than one allergen? *Contact Dermatitis* 21:122-124, 1989.

Epstein E: *Primula* contact dermatitis: an easily overlooked diagnosis, *Cutis* 45:411-416, 1990.

Fernàndez de Corrè L, Leanizbarrutia I, Munoz D: Contact dermatitis from *Primula obconica* hance, *Contact Dermatitis* 16:195-197, 1987.

Hausen BM, Heitsch H, Borrmann B, et al: Structure-activity relationships in allergic contact dermatitis. I. Studies on the influence of side-chain length with derivatives of primin, *Contact Dermatitis* 33:12-16, 1995.

Ingber A, Mennè T: Primin standard patch testing: 5 years' experience, *Contact Dermatitis* 23:15-19, 1990.

Krebs M, Christensen LP: 2-methoxy-6-pentyl-1,4-dihydroxy-benzene (miconidin) from *Primula obconica:* a possible allergen? *Contact Dermatitis* 33:90-93, 1995.

Logan RA, White IR: *Primula* dermatitis: prevalence, detection, and outcome, *Contact Dermatitis* 19:68-69, 1988.

Mowad CM: Routine testing for *Primula obconica:* is it useful in the United States? *Am J Contact Dermat* 9:231-233, 1998.

Tabar AI, Quirce S, Garcia BE et al: *Primula* dermatitis: versatility in its clinical presentation and the advantages of patch tests with synthetic primin, *Contact Dermatitis* 30:47-48, 1994.

Virgili A, Corazza M: Unusual primin dermatitis, *Contact Dermatitis* 24:63-64, 1991.

RAGWEED

Definition

Ragweed is a common aggressive pioneer weed found widely in North America. It is a member of the Compositae family of plants and belongs to the genus *Ambrosia.* The incidence of allergic contact dermatitis due to ragweed appears to be declining in recent years. Patch testing can be accomplished with extracts of short and giant ragweed.

Clinical Aspects

Allergic contact dermatitis from ragweed is due to sesquiterpene lactones that are found in the plant. Several species have caused ragweed dermatitis, including short and giant ragweeds. The dermatitis is chronic and lichenified, predominantly affecting adult male farmers and rural workers. Its distribution mimics a photo-dermatitis affecting the exposed skin of the hands, forearms, neck, and face but also affects areas that are spared in photodermatitis: the upper eyelids and the retroauricular and submental skin. In contrast to allergic conjunctivitis and allergic respiratory disease caused by ragweed pollen during the late summer and fall, ragweed dermatitis occurs during the entire growing season from spring through fall. It is initially limited to this time of year, but with chronicity the dermatitis becomes perennial and disseminated. Contact dermatitis can occur directly from the plant or from fomites carrying the allergen, such as hay, cotton, grain, flour, boots, hatbands, and clothes.

Allergic contact dermatitis due to ragweed should be considered in patients suspected of having photodermatitis, especially if the upper eyelids and the retroauricular and submental skin are affected. Patch testing is best done with ragweed extracts.

BIBLIOGRAPHY

Mitchell JC, Roy AK, Dupuis G et al: Allergic contact dermatitis from ragweeds (*Ambrosia* species): the role of sesquiterpene lactones, *Arch Dermatol* 104:73-76, 1971.

Schmidt RJ: Compositae, *Clin Dermatol* 4:46-61, 1986.

Shelmire B: Contact dermatitis from weeds: patch testing with oleoresins, *JAMA* 113:1085-1090, 1939.

TULIP

Definition

Tulips are a favorite spring flower for formal bedding gardens, window boxes, and cut flowers. They are a member of the family Liliaceae and genus *Tulipa*. Despite being short-lived and producing a scentless flower, the tulip is cherished because of its elegant, stately beauty. Allergic contact dermatitis to tulips is predominantly seen in the flower bulb industry. Patch testing is done with tuliposide A (at 0.1%) or α-methylene-γ-butyrolactone (0.01%) in petrolatum or with portions of the white outer bulb.

> **Tuliposide A, the allergen in tulips, is also found in *Alstroemeria* species. Patch testing can be done with tuliposide A, α-methylene-γ-butyrolactone, or with the outer, white epidermis of the tulip bulb.**

Clinical Aspects

Allergic contact dermatitis to tulip bulbs is known as "tulip fingers" and has been reported in workers who have extensive direct contact with tulip bulbs during digging, peeling, sorting, and packaging. Tulip fingers characteristically involves the fingertips and periungual skin with chronic, erythematous, fissured, scaling, painful plaques (Plate 70). An investigation of an American bulb distributor revealed a high sensitization rate of 56%. Five of nine workers had allergic contact dermatitis that was due to tulip bulbs that they sorted and packed (Gette and Marks, 1990). In a Swedish nursery where mainly tulips were grown, 9 (17.6%) of 51 workers were sensitive to tulips and had allergic contact dermatitis.

Tuliposide A is the major allergen found in the white epidermis of tulip bulbs and also in the stem, flower, pistils, and leaves of the tulip. Florists who handle cut tulip flowers are at risk of developing allergic contact dermatitis. Tuliposide A is not unique to *Tulipa* species but is found in other plants, particularly *Alstroemeria* species. This is particularly important, since the genus *Alstroemeria* is a common cause of allergic contact dermatitis in florists. Thus individuals developing a sensitivity to tulip bulbs can react to *Alstroemeria* species and vice versa.

Allergic contact dermatitis, a type IV, delayed-type hypersensitivity, is the most common allergic reaction to tulip bulbs. Besides tulip fingers, a diffuse dermatitis called tulip fire has been reported. Tulip fire is thought to be secondary to airborne particles of the outer layers of the bulb. In addition, type I, immediate hypersensitivity reactions can occur. Symptoms of contact urticaria, rhinitis, hoarseness, and dyspnea have been described in a florist during cutting of tulips. Scratch test reactions with extracts from tulip bulbs and stems were positive.

Horticultural workers sometimes suspect that a pesticide is the cause of their skin eruptions. An outbreak of face and arm dermatitis among half of the employees in a tulip bulb processing company was found to be allergic contact dermatitis to a newly introduced fungicide, fluazinam, not tulips.

BIBLIOGRAPHY

Bruze M, Björkner B, Hellström AC: Occupational dermatoses in nursery workers, *Am J Contact Dermat* 7:100-103, 1996.

Bruynzeel DP, De Boer EM, Brouwer EJ et al: Dermatitis in bulb growers, *Contact Dermatitis* 29:11-15, 1993.

Bruynzeel DP, Tafelkruijer J, Wilks MF: Contact dermatitis due to a new fungicide used in the tulip bulb industry, *Contact Dermatitis* 33:8-11, 1995.

Christensen LP, Kristiansen K: Isolation and quantification of tuliposides and tulipalins in tulips *(Tulipa)* by high-performance liquid chromatography, *Contact Dermatitis* 40:300-309, 1999.

Gette MT, Marks JG: Tulip fingers, *Arch Dermatol* 126:203-205, 1990.

Hausen BM: Airborne contact dermatitis caused by tulip bulbs, *J Am Acad Dermatol* 7:500-503, 1982.

Lahti A: Contact urticaria and respiratory symptoms from tulips and lilies, *Contact Dermatitis* 14:317-319, 1986.

Slob A: Tulip allergens in *Alstroemeria* and some other Liliiflorae, *Phytochemistry* 12:811-815, 1973.

Verspyck Mijnssen GAW: Pathogenesis and causative agent of "tulip finger," *Br J Dermatol* 81:737-745, 1969.

Welker WH, Rappaport BZ: Dermatitis due to tulip bulbs, *J Allergy* 3:317, 1932.

WILD FEVERFEW

Definition

Wild feverfew, *Parthenium hysterophorus,* is one of the weeds in the family Compositae that causes allergic contact dermatitis. It grows in cultivated land and wastelands of North and South America. It has caused an epidemic of allergic contact dermatitis in India after being accidentally introduced via imported wheat from the United States. Allergic contact dermatitis to wild feverfew can be

Benzalkonium chloride is used as a preservative in medications dispensed in multidose vials for injection, including sterile saline, and is used in the cold sterilization of medical and dental instruments. It is present in some plaster of Paris and is used in the dye, fabric, metallurgy, and agricultural industries.

Despite extensive usage of benzalkonium chloride, the risk of sensitization is considered to be low in general. It has been reported to cause conjunctivitis and periorbital dermatitis, cheilitis and stomatitis, and dermatitis around treated wounds.

It has caused occupational contact dermatitis in health care workers from handling disinfectants, topical preparations, and cold sterilized instruments. An endotracheal tube cold sterilized with benzalkonium chloride has induced an unusual contact tracheitis. Occupational contact dermatitis in persons involved in cleaning procedures using detergents that contain benzalkonium chloride (e.g., floor cleaner, cook, or farm worker) has been reported. Cases of airborne dermatitis from this chemical have also been reported. Occupational asthma caused by prolonged exposure to a cleaning solution containing benzalkonium chloride has been described earlier.

Cross-reactivity may occur with other quaternary ammonium compounds including *cetrimide, desqualinium chloride, cetalkonium chloride, benzethonium chloride,* and *chloroallylhexaminium chloride.*

Generalized dermatitis may occur in individuals who are sensitized to quaternary ammonium compounds when they are administered chemically related systemic medications. These include *tetraethylammonium chloride, decamethonium bromide,* and *hexadimethrine bromide.*

The benzalkonium chloride patch test result must be read with care, since even a 0.1% concentration may produce irritant responses. It may also cause delayed irritation and patch test reactions increasing in intensity with time. Therefore dilution series should always be used to confirm the allergic nature of a positive patch test reaction to this chemical. A repeated open application test (ROAT) can be useful to determine its clinical relevance.

BIBLIOGRAPHY

Andersen KE, Rycroft RJG: Recommended patch test concentrations for preservatives, biocides, and antimicrobials, *Contact Dermatitis* 25:1-18, 1991.

Bernstein JA, Stauder T, Bernstein DI, Bernstein IL: A combined respiratory and cutaneous hypersensitivity syndrome induced by work exposure to quaternary amines, *J Allergy Clin Immunol* 94:257-259, 1994.

Corazza M, Virgili A: Airborne allergic contact dermatitis from benzalkonium chloride, *Contact Dermatitis* 28:195-196, 1993.

Fuchs T et al: Benzalkonium chloride: a relevant contact allergen or irritant? *Hautarzt* 44:699-702, 1993.

Kanerva L, Jolanki R, Estlander T: Occupational allergic contact dermatitis from benzalkonium chloride, *Contact Dermatitis* 42:357, 2000.

Klein GF, Sepp N, Fritsch P: Allergic reactions to benzalkonium chloride? Do the use test! *Contact Dermatitis* 25:269-270, 1991.

Rustemeyer T, Pilz B, Frosch PJ: Contact allergies in medical and paramedical professions, *Hautarzt* 45:834-844, 1994.

Stanford D, Georgouras K: Allergic contact dermatitis from benzalkonium chloride in plaster of Paris, *Contact Dermatitis* 35:371-72, 1996.

CAPTAN

Definition

Captan (*N*-trichloromethylthio-4-cyclohexene-1,2-dicarboximide) is widely used as a fungicide and pesticide in agriculture and floristry. It is also used as an antiseborrheic and antibacterial in personal care products, particularly those designed for hair. Captan is also used in veterinary medicine as a topical treatment for ticks and fleas.

Clinical Aspects

Captan is primarily used as a fungicide in the agricultural industry. In such a setting captan has produced occupational allergic contact dermatitis, usually in an airborne or exposed-site distribution.

Captan under the synonyms Vancide 89 and Dangard is used as a bacteriostat, a preservative, and an antiseborrheic in cosmetics, particularly in shampoos and hair treatments. Selsun, Selsun Blue, Capitrol, and salon products, now or in the past, have contained captan. In such products captan achieved a usage level equal to one 30th of the level for quaternium-15 in the United States in 1990. Cases of occupational allergic contact dermatitis in hairdressers have been described.

> **Captan is used as a plant and animal pesticide and as a component of antiseborrheic shampoos and salon hair products.**

EXPOSURE LIST ▶ **CAPTAN**

Synonyms and Other Names

Dangard	*N*-trichloromethylthio-4-cyclohexene-1,2-dicarboximide
Merpan	Vancide
Orthocide-406	Vancide 89
SR-406	Vancide 89 RE

Uses

Captan is used as a plant fungicide, a veterinary flea and tick treatment, and a cosmetic preservative and antiseborrheic in the following types of products:
1. Shampoos
2. Hair tonics and creams
3. Plant and fruit sprays and powders
4. Animal flea and tick sprays

Prevention

Patients who are allergic to captan should be instructed to read the ingredient lists of all cosmetics, especially those used on hair, and avoid products containing captan or labeled with the names listed previously. Animal flea and tick treatment products should be checked for the presence of captan. Agricultural workers may be exposed to captan pesticides that are used to treat fruits, vegetables, and other plants.

May be duplicated for use in clinical practice. From Marks JG Jr, Elsner P, DeLeo VA: *Contact and occupational dermatology*, ed 2, St Louis, 1997, Mosby.

Textile finish dermatitis is caused primarily by formaldehyde related resins, which are used as additives to improve the wrinkle resistance, strength, and feel of the finished garment. These agents are used primarily in blends of natural and synthetic fibers but may be used in fabric made of pure natural fibers as well. The allergy induced by these agents may be due to formaldehyde that is released from the resin in the fabric or by the resin itself. About 70% of patients with textile resin allergy will have a positive patch test to formaldehyde as tested in the standard tray. In the others the resin itself is the allergen, and such patients must be tested to the resin to confirm the allergy. One such resin that appears to be a good screening test is *ethyleneurea/melamine formaldehyde resin 5% in petrolatum.*

Textile dye allergy is much less common than resin-related allergy. Most of the dyes that cause sensitization are disperse azo and anthraquinone dyes, and they are used primarily to dye synthetic fibers. Since such dyes are chemically related to para-phenylene diamine, that allergen in the standard tray may act as a screen for textile dye allergy. It is, however, not sufficient in detecting most textile dye–sensitive individuals. Presently, an additional second screening agent to be recommended is either Disperse Blue 106 or 124.

When textile allergy is suspected, it is recommended that samples of clothing be tested as well as the standard tray and the two allergens listed previously. The sample of cloth should be soaked in water or saline for about 15 minutes and may be left in place as a patch test for longer than the usual 48 hours (72 to 96 hours). In addition, when dye allergy is suspected, the fabric may be soaked in warmed ethanol for 60 minutes before application (Reitschel and Fowler, 2001).

ETHYLENEUREA/MELAMINE FORMALDEHYDE RESIN
Definition

Ethyleneurea/melamine formaldehyde resin is one of a large group of fabric finishing agents used to treat natural fibers and natural-synthetic blends to make the finished textile wrinkle- and shrink-resistant. This group of agents is derived from urea and melamine formaldehyde polycondensation products that are polymerized within the fibers. Ethyleneurea/melamine formaldehyde resin is tested at 5% in petrolatum. In the 1996 to 1998 testing period for the North American Contact Dermatitis Group, 7.2% of individuals tested had positive reactions to this antigen. The disease produced by this agent is sometimes referred to as *permanent press* or *durable press dermatitis.*

Clinical Aspects

In the 1930s clothing manufacturers developed formaldehyde-derived chemicals to treat cotton and other natural fibers to make them stronger and more shrink- and wrinkle-resistant. The majority of these agents were derived from urea and melamine formaldehyde condensation products. Since that time, improvement in the technology has led to the development of a large number of these methylol formaldehyde–containing chemicals. They are used primarily in the production of cloth from natural fibers and natural-synthetic blends.

> **Formaldehyde is released from treated textiles, and either the formaldehyde or the complete resin can induce sensitization in certain individuals.**

The dermatitis produced is usually a subacute patchy dermatitis that may resemble nummular or asteototic eczema. Such patients may also be misdiagnosed as having adult-onset atopic eczema or neurodermatitis. The eruption usually spares the hands and face and may be accentuated in areas where clothing has tighter contact with the skin, like the neck, thighs, and axillary lines. Patients tend to be older, and men and women are similarly affected. Itching may be severe.

EXPOSURE LIST ▶ **ETHYLENEUREA/MELAMINE FORMALDEHYDE RESIN**

Synonyms and Other Names
Fixapret AC

Uses
Ethyleneurea/melamine formaldehyde resin is one of a number of textile additives that are used in fabrics. These agents are used to decrease wrinkling of fabrics used for clothing and other textiles like bed linens. Ethyleneurea/melamine formaldehyde resin is used in the following:
1. Clothing
2. Bedding
3. Fabrics

Prevention
A positive patch test reaction to this agent suggests a textile or fabric allergy. This allergen may also be positive in patients who have allergy to other formaldehyde-containing agents like preservatives in creams and lotions. If the patient does not exhibit dermatitis in areas of fabric contact, he or she is probably not being affected by this allergy.

If an individual has a clothing dermatitis caused by this agent, the following steps should be taken to avoid the allergen:
1. Wear loose-fitting garments.
2. Wash all new clothing and bed linens at least twice before usage.
3. Avoid:
   - Permanent-press garments
   - Rayon blends
   - Corduroy
   - Blended fabrics (cotton-polyester)
   - Shrink-proof wool
4. Wear 100%:
   - Silk
   - Linen
   - Wool
   - Denim
   - Nylon
   - Polyester
   - Mercerized cotton
5. If you must wear suspicious clothing, do so over silk or nylon underwear.

The clinical picture may be confusing, since some of these individuals will also be reactive to formaldehyde-releasing preservatives in their personal care products and cosmetics. In such cases the face and hands may also be involved.

Patients suspected of having this problem should be tested to formaldehyde and ethyleneurea/melamine formaldehyde resin, which are thought to be the best screening agents for resin allergy. The majority of patients will be sensitive to formaldehyde. Other screening allergens include urea formaldehyde resin, tetramethylol acetelenediurea formaldehyde resin, dimethylol dihydroxyethelene urea formaldehyde resin, and dimethylolpropylene urea formaldehyde resin.

In addition to resin allergens and formaldehyde, it is sometimes recommended that patients' garments be tested. Small pieces of fabric from suspected clothing can be soaked in water or saline for 15 minutes before being applied in a Finn chamber. False negative reactions do occur, but the possibility of a positive reaction may be enhanced by leaving these patches on for 72 to 96 hours.

Allergic individuals may also have to avoid certain cosmetics and medicated creams that contain formaldehyde-releasing preservatives. The physician should discuss this with the allergic individual.

BIBLIOGRAPHY

Fowler JF, Skinner S, Belsito D: Allergic contact dermatitis from formaldehyde resin in permanent-press clothing, *J Am Acad Dermatol* 27:962-963, 1992.

Marks JG, Belsito DV, DeLeo VA: North American Contact Dermatitis Group standard tray patch test results: 1996 to 1998, *Arch Dermatol* 136(2):272-273, 2000.

Rietschel RL, Fowler JF: *Fisher's contact dermatitis,* ed 5, Philadelphia, 2001, Lippincott Williams & Wilkins.

DISPERSE BLUE DYES 106 AND 124

Definition

Disperse dyes are azo and anthraquinones, which are used primarily to dye synthetic fabrics, especially polyesters. Disperse Blue dyes 106 and 124 are the most commonly used screening dye allergens. Both allergens are tested at a 1% concentration in petrolatum. In a recent Canadian study of individuals with suspected textile dermatitis, 82.5% and 80% of the patients found to be allergic to textile dyes reacted to Disperse Blue 106 and Disperse Blue 124, respectively.

Clinical Aspects

Textiles for all uses have been dyed to enhance their appeal since ancient times. Chemicals used for that purpose encompass many different structural classes and are usually classified according to the process used to apply the dye to the textile. Disperse dyes are the agents most commonly involved in producing allergic contact dermatitis. Chemically these agents are azoic anthraquinones and nitroarylamines.

> **Disperse dyes are used primarily to dye synthetic fabrics, especially polyesters and acetates.**

EXPOSURE LIST ▷ **DISPERSE BLUE DYES 106 AND 124**

Synonyms and Other Names
None

Uses
Disperse Blue dyes 106 and 124 are chemicals added to textiles and fabrics to enhance their visual appeal. These two dyes are used primarily to dye polyester and acetate textiles, but they can be used to dye color blended and natural fabrics as well. Since they are blue dyes, they are found in fabrics that are blue, but they are also found in any dark color like black or brown and may also be found in lighter green and violet/purple shades. They are used in the following:
1. Clothing
2. Bedding
3. Fabrics

Prevention
A positive patch test to either of these agents suggests a textile or clothing allergy.
   If an individual has a clothing dermatitis caused by these dyes, the following steps should be taken to avoid the allergen:
1. Avoid:
   - Garments, especially those made from pure polyester and acetate and polyester and acetate blends, that are colored blue, other dark colors like black and brown, and green and violet/purple.
   - Synthetic spandex/lycra exercise clothing in the colors listed above.
   - Nylon stockings, especially dark colors.
2. Wear loose-fitting garments.
3. Wash all new clothing and bed linens at least twice before usage
4. Remove dark-colored liners from clothing and have them replaced with white liners.
5. Wear 100% natural-based fabrics like silk, wool, linen, and cotton.
6. Wear 100% white silk long-sleeved underwear and slips if outerwear is suspected to be a problem and cannot be avoided.
7. Wear Levi Strauss 501 blue jeans, which do not usually cause dermatitis in dye-sensitive individuals.

The most common Disperse dyes found to cause allergic contact dermatitis are Disperse Blue 106 and 124; Disperse Red 1, 17, and 43; Disperse Orange 3; and Disperse Yellow 3.

Patients with dye dermatitis usually present with an acute or subacute dermatitis involving the axillary folds and waistband areas, the upper inner thighs and arms, the buttocks, popliteal fossae, and the genital and perineal areas. A more generalized dermatitis can occur, but the presentation is different from the chronic indolent picture seen in clothing dermatitis caused by resin allergy. This is partly because dye allergens would be expected to be present in fewer pieces of clothing in an individual's wardrobe, whereas resin allergens would be more widespread.

Women are usually more likely to develop allergies to these agents than men, and the most common fabrics involved are polyester and acetate liners of women's clothing.

There is no single screening agent for all dye allergies. Para-phenylene diamine has been suggested but will be positive in less than 30% of dye-sensitive individuals. Disperse Blue dyes 106 or 124 should be used with any patient suspected of having a textile dye allergy.

When dye allergy is suspected, it may be necessary to test the suspected fabric, but this may yield false-negative results. Patches may need to be left in place for more than the standard 48 hours.

The most common dyes responsible for contact allergy in the 1990s were the Disperse Blue dyes 106 and 124, which caused a mini-epidemic in Canada. They have been reported to cause problems when used to dye polyester blouses, underwear, pants, suits, swimsuits, pantyhose, shoulder pads, velvet leggings and bodysuits, and particularly liners for dresses, suits, and pants.

> **Patch test responses to Disperse Blue dyes 106 and 124 may be delayed for up to 7 to 10 days.**

BIBLIOGRAPHY

Hatch KL, Maibach HI: Textile dye dermatitis, *J Am Acad Dermatol* 32:631-639, 1995.

Pratt M, Taraska T: Disperse blue dyes 106 and 124 are common causes of textile dermatitis and should serve as screening allergens for this condition, *Am J Contact Dermat* 11:30-41, 2000.

Reitschel RI, Fowler JF: *Fisher's contact dermatitis,* ed 5, Philadelphia, 2001, Lippincott Williams & Wilkins.

PART III

Occupational Skin Disease

hand eczema probably also contributes to the poor prognosis once it develops. Despite avoidance of irritants and allergens, reactivation or exacerbation of atopic hand dermatitis can result in prolonged, severe dermatitis, even with the best possible medical care. Other characteristics of the atopic individual such as xerotic skin, inherent pruritus, dysfunctional sweating, and a high carriage rate of *Staphylococcus aureus* also contribute to the development of occupational skin disease in these individuals.

Psoriasis, Acne, and Stasis Dermatitis

The other cutaneous disorders previously mentioned may predispose the worker to the development of occupational skin disease. For workers with psoriasis, aggravating factors at work such as repeated skin trauma can precipitate a psoriatic lesion—Koebner's phenomenon. This may be disabling for workers with psoriasis of the palms and soles who are required to perform manual tasks with their hands or have prolonged walking and standing. Occupational acne occurs in those who have exposure to cutting oils and greases or work in a hot, humid environment. A greater amount of body hair has been cited as a predisposing factor for developing acne and folliculitis. For individuals with venous insufficiency and stasis dermatitis, jobs with prolonged standing are detrimental to workers and predispose them to the development of stasis ulcers.

Skin Color

Fair skin is an obvious predisposing risk factor for the development of skin cancer in individuals with outdoor occupations such as farming and sailing. In addition, the propensity for fair-skinned individuals to develop skin cancer is increased even more in jobs with exposure to sunlight plus phototoxic chemicals such as pitch and tar. Black skin appears to be less susceptible than white skin to contact irritants and allergens. Dark skin is better protected from the damage of ultraviolet light, but the development of keloids after injury is a potential problem in the workplace.

Age

A host factor that seems to predispose to the development of occupational skin disease is aging skin, which appears to be less resistant to injury. On the other hand, the younger, inexperienced workers are at risk for developing occupational skin disease because they are less cautious in avoiding hazards and have not become acclimated or hardened to chemical contactants within their workplace. Thus a bimodal distribution of occupational dermatitis is seen, with the youngest and oldest workers being most affected.

Hygiene

Personal hygiene is an important indirect host factor in the development of skin disease. The worker who neglects washing away irritating chemicals or who has poor personal hygienic habits is highly susceptible to developing occupational skin disease. The employer, however, has a responsibility to provide protective clothing, laundering facilities when necessary, and adequate washing facilities for the worker. Education of the worker by the employer concerning hygienic measures and avoidance of overzealous cleansing is often necessary.

JOB-RELATED FACTORS

Irritants

Irritant contact dermatitis is generally considered to cause approximately three fourths of cases of occupational contact dermatitis. The proportion of irritant contact dermatitis, however, varies widely in studies of occupational dermatitis. Although irritant contact dermatitis is the most common cause of occupational skin disease, it is the least understood and reported because of its multiple forms, lack of a diagnostic test, and multiple mechanisms involved in its production. The diagnosis of irritant contact dermatitis is primarily based on a history of exposure to a known irritant and negative patch test results to exclude contact allergy. The combination of physicochemical properties of the irritant, exposure conditions, and host factors determines the degree of irritation. The clinical appearance can vary greatly from painful erythema, edema, vesiculation, and necrosis to stinging and pruritic erythema, dryness, scaling, and fissured patches and plaques. Irritants may be strong, moderate, or weak. Lists of occupational irritants and higher-risk occupations for irritant contact dermatitis are provided in Tables 12-2 and 12-3.

Table 12-2

Occupational Irritants

Type	Examples
Acids	Sulfuric, hydrochloric, nitric, chromic, hydrofluoric, salicylic
Alkalis	Potassium and sodium hydroxide, calcium oxide, hydroxide
Animal products	Enzymes
Metalworking fluids	Water-based coolants
Organic solvents	Benzene, toluene, acetone, methyl ethyl ketone, acrylonitrile, carbon bisulfide
Oxidizing agents	Benzoyl peroxide, sodium hypochlorite
Petroleum products	Solvents, gasoline, grease
Physical agents	Fiberglass, paper, metal dust, abrasive materials
Plants	Dumbcane, buttercup, croton, May apple, onion
Reducing agents	Phenols, hydrazines, thioglycolates, aldehydes
Soaps and detergents	Dishwashing liquid, shampoo, cleaning agents
Water	

Table 12-3

High-Risk Occupations for Irritant Contact Dermatitis

Agricultural workers	Housekeeping workers
Bakers	Mechanics
Bartenders	Medical and dental personnel
Butchers	Metalworkers
Construction workers	Painters
Food preparers	Printers
Florists	Roofers
Hairdressers	Rubber, leather, and other manufacturing jobs
Horticulturalists	Textile workers

The diagnosis of occupationally induced irritant contact dermatitis requires the following: (1) exposure to a known occupational irritant, (2) improvement away from work, and (3) negative patch test reactions to relevant workplace allergens.

Strong irritants are easily recognized because they cause rapid cutaneous injury that is manifested by strong burning and followed by cutaneous inflammation. Strong irritants include ethylene oxide, hydrofluoric acid, and wet cement. *Ethylene oxide* is used for gas sterilization of medical items such as anesthesia masks, medical devices, and surgical gowns and drapes. Burns in hospital workers and patients have occurred after incompletely aerated masks, gowns, and sheets were used. *Hydrofluoric acid* is an extremely cytotoxic agent used widely in the electronics and semiconductor industries. The deep, throbbing, excruciating pain of hydrofluoric acid burns is an important harbinger of potential deep-tissue injury to nerves, blood vessels, tendons, and bone. The symptoms may initially be out of proportion to the observed injury. These patients require close follow-up after first aid with copious water lavage and topical neutralization agents. Severe exposure requires repeated calcium gluconate infiltrations or infusions. Prolonged contact with *wet cement,* especially under occlusion, is another cause of acute irritant contact dermatitis that can result in severe burns from the highly alkaline calcium oxide formed when water is added to dry cement. Within 12 to 24 hours, deep necrotic ulcers appear and can lead to deep, disfiguring scars.

Mild to moderate irritants cause most of the cutaneous problems. The variability and frequent nonreproducibility of mild to moderate irritants to produce dermatitis make full appreciation and understanding of these irritant reactions difficult. The nonimmunologic inflammatory reaction, which often is insidious, results from multiple exposures. Because the dermatitis results from the cumulative effect of multiple minor skin irritations, the worker may not be cognizant of the cause of this reaction. In addition, previously mentioned endogenous factors such as atopic dermatitis can significantly contribute to the development of irritant contact dermatitis from mild to moderate irritants. The distinction between mild to moderate irritancy and allergy is not possible on morphologic criteria, on either gross or histologic examination. The diagnosis of irritant contact dermatitis is made clinically by taking into consideration the nature of the chemical and the circumstances of exposure. Patch testing is done to exclude allergic contact dermatitis. The most common skin irritants are solvents, soaps, detergents, fiberglass, metalworking fluids, water, and a number of other natural and synthetic compounds. For example, a single washing with a surfactant or soap can cause marked dehydration and delipidation of the stratum corneum. Further damage to the skin is caused by repetitive washing, and extended time (weeks) is needed for complete healing of the irritant skin reaction.

Irritants cause approximately 75% of occupationally induced contact dermatitis. Allergens are responsible for 25%.

Allergens

Allergic contact dermatitis is less common than irritation and accounts for approximately 25% of occupational contact dermatitis. The morphologic appearance of allergic contact dermatitis is typically indistinguishable from irritant dermatitis with the exception of acute tissue necrosis from strong irritants. Many chemicals are both allergens and irritants. For example, at a high concentration methylchloroisothiazolinone/methylisothiazolinone is an irritant, whereas at a lower, subirritating concentration it is an allergen. This can be troublesome, particularly when patch testing, because some allergens such as formaldehyde are patch tested at a near-irritant level. The ability of chemicals to sensitize is quite variable: some are strong sensitizers, and others weak. Strong sensitizers include poison ivy and oak oleoresin and dinitrochlorobenzene. Weak sensitizers include the parabens and high-molecular-weight chemicals such as polyurethanes. The diagnosis of allergic contact dermatitis can be positively made only by patch testing. The importance of diagnosing allergic contact dermatitis is paramount in the management and prevention of occupational skin disease.

Infections

A number of infectious agents are responsible for occupational skin disease. With public health measures the importance of many infections has greatly diminished in the general population. Their impact, however, can still be significant in selected occupational groups such as health care workers, farmers, military personnel, and forestry workers.

A number of *bacterial* infections can have an occupational origin. Staphylococcal and streptococcal infections occur in construction and farm workers, meat packers, and workers in other jobs in which minor lacerations, abrasions, puncture wounds, or burns may become secondarily infected and cause impetigo, cellulitis, furuncles, and abscesses. Anthrax in the United States is almost always cutaneous and is found in occupations in which workers handle imported goat hair, wool, and hides contaminated with spores from the bacterium *Bacillus anthracis.* Fishermen and butchers are at risk of the *Erysipelothrix rhusiopathiae* infection erysipeloid from infected fish, pork, and poultry. Atypical *Mycobacterium* species infections are most common in workers in aquatic environments such as people who clean fish tanks and fishermen. Tuberculosis of the skin that was acquired through inoculation of *Mycobacterium tuberculosis* as an occupational risk was previously seen in pathologists and morgue attendants. Other occupationally induced bacterial infections include brucellosis, tularemia, glanders, and cat scratch disease.

Viral infections are common occupationally acquired diseases. Herpes simplex infections among health care workers, particularly dental workers and others who have frequent contact with the oral cavity, are prone to develop an infection of the fingers, herpetic whitlow. More recently, with the emergence of the human immunodeficiency virus (HIV), acquisition of infection from body fluids and accidental puncture wounds is particularly worrisome in medical personnel. Orf, or ecthyma contagiosum, infects sheep and goats and is readily transmitted to their handlers. Milker's nodule is a paravaccinia virus infection among dairy farmers and veterinarians who have direct contact with infected teats and udders of cattle. Viral warts occur with increased frequency in butchers and poultry slaughterers.

PLANT INSPECTION

NAME: DATE:
ADDRESS: PHONE:
MANAGER: FAX:

1.   MANUFACTURING PROCESS

     Outline the manufacturing process with an understanding of the technology and division of labor.

2.   WALK-THROUGH AND EXAMINATION OF EMPLOYEES

     During the walk-through, examine exposed areas of the worker's skin, and note the number of
     workers in each department who have dermatitis.

     Job—Department   # Workers   # Dermatitis

3.   GENERAL WORKING CONDITIONS

     Temperature_____   Humidity_____   Odor_____
     Cleanliness_____
     Chemicals properly stored and dispensed_____
     Closed vs. open systems_____

4.   PROTECTIVE CLOTHING—WASHROOM FACILITIES

     Available?
     Used and properly worn?
     Moisturizers_____
     Soaps_____

5.   ALLERGENS AND IRRITANTS (ESPECIALLY SUSPECTED OFFENDERS)

     Material Safety Data Sheets:

     Name of Chemical   Location in Plant

6.   PLANT DISPENSARY

     Discuss problem with the nurse, hygienist, or plant doctor.
     Review medical histories and medicines dispensed. Take an occupational history and physical
     examination of a couple of workers.

7.   SUMMARY—CONCLUSIONS
     Further investigators?—toxicologists, NIOSH, etc.
     Further testing?—patch tests, laboratory screen, etc.
     Preventive measures?

FIGURE 13-1
Outline of the plant survey.

chemist. Enough time should be allowed to inspect the workplace in a deliber-
ate, unhurried manner. We have found that 3 hours is usually adequate. Since the
processes and chemicals are usually new to the physician, do not be afraid to ask
simple questions. A vague or poorly understood manufacturing operation can easily lead to incorrect conclusions. The type of assistance provided depends very

much on the size of the factory. Large manufacturers will have a number of individuals available, including full-time medical personnel or a director of health and safety.

The initial portion of the plant inspection should be used to understand the technology and division of labor. This should be accomplished before the walk-through so that the examining physician has an overview of the industrial operation, materials used, and perceived problems, along with actions that have been taken to date. The walk-through of the plant can then proceed with a tour guide who is knowledgeable about the work process and materials contacted. It is helpful to tour the plant in the order in which the manufacturing process occurs, starting with the delivery of raw materials and finishing with the manufactured product. This reinforces the initial overview of the manufacturing process that was given before the actual walk-through.

During the *walk-through* a number of observations are made. The general working conditions such as tidiness, storage of chemicals, and ambient conditions are noted. The exposed skin of the workers can be briefly examined for the presence of dermatitis. Their jobs and the number of workers doing those jobs are recorded. The availability of protective clothing and whether it is properly worn must be noted. Are washroom facilities readily available, and what types of cleansers and moisturizers are used? The chemicals used by the workers should be recorded, along with their location in the plant and the material safety data sheets collected. Often, the number of materials becomes overwhelming, so only offending chemicals that are suspected by the workers or management should be investigated initially.

After the walk-through, selected workers with dermatitis may be interviewed and examined in more detail following the outline of the occupational history and physical examination. This can be accomplished in the plant dispensary or possibly a conference room. A more detailed examination of these workers may reveal their eruptions to be nonoccupational. Often workers perceive noneczematous conditions such as acne and dermatophyte infections to be work-related when in fact they are nonoccupational.

> **During the walk-through, leading questions and premature conclusions should be avoided.**

A preliminary verbal summary may be given to the plant management, but a final written report should be made. The written report should follow the outline of the plant inspect and describe the manufacturing processes, the walk-through examination of employees, the general working conditions, the protective clothing and washroom facilities, a description of the suspected offending chemicals and, where applicable, a more detailed examination of selected workers. Treatment and preventive measures may be recommended or further investigations suggested, such as an epidemiologic study that establishes a case definition, a target population, a characterization of the outbreak, and a statistical analysis. There are considerable resources locally, statewide, and federally to assist in an in-depth investigation of the workplace.

BIBLIOGRAPHY

Adams RM: Panels of allergens for specific occupations, *J Am Acad Dermatol* 21:869-874, 1989.

Adams RM: Plant survey inspection. In Adams RM, editor: *Occupational skin disease*, ed 2, Philadelphia, 1990, WB Saunders.

Carmichael AJ, Foulds IS: Performing a factory visit, *Clin Exper Dermatol* 18:208-210, 1993.

DeGroot AC: *Patch testing: test concentrations and vehicles for* 3700 *chemicals,* ed 2, Amsterdam, 1994, Elsevier.

Diepgen TL, Fartasch M, Hornstein OP: Evaluation and relevance of atopic basic and minor features in patients with atopic dermatitis and in the general population, *Acta Derm Venereol (Suppl)* 144:50-54, 1989.

Freeman S: Diagnosis and differential diagnosis. In Adams RM, editor: *Occupational skin disease*, ed 2, Philadelphia, 1990, WB Saunders.

Fregert S: Patch testing with isolated and identified substances in products: basis for prevention, *J Am Acad Dermatol* 21:857-860, 1989.

Hinnen U, Elsner P: Irritancy exposure assessment in metal worker, *Curr Probl Dermatol* 22:67-71, 1995.

Lookingbill DP: Yield from a complete skin examination: findings in 1157 new dermatology patients, *J Am Acad Dermatol* 18:31-37, 1988.

Marrakchi S, Maibach HI: What is occupational contact dermatitis? an operational definition, *Dermatol Clin* 12:477-487, 1994.

Mathias CGT: Contact dermatitis and workers' compensation: criteria for establishing occupational causation and aggravation, *J Am Acad Dermatol* 20:842-848, 1989.

Mitchell JC: Documentation for workers' compensation dermatitis, *Contact Dermatitis* 9:430-432, 1983.

Moshell AN: Occupational skin disease: where are the dermatologists? *J Am Acad Dermatol* 4:729-732, 1981.

Rietschel RL: Patch testing in occupational hand dermatitis, *Dermatol Clin* 6:43-46, 1988.

Rycroft RJG: False reactions to nonstandard patch tests, *Semin Dermatol* 5:225-230, 1986.

Rycroft RJG: Occupational dermatoses in perspective, *Lancet* 2:24-26, 1980.

The Occupational and Environmental Health Committee of the American Lung Association of San Diego and Imperial Counties, San Diego, California: Taking the occupational history, *Ann Intern Med* 99:641-651, 1983.

Tong DW: Conducting a factory or plant visit, *Australas J Dermatol* 36:129-132, 1995.

CHAPTER 14

Management of Occupational Dermatitis

PREVENTION
    Hazardous material identification
    High-risk population identification
    Hazard control
        Employer
        Worker
        Government
        Health care
THERAPY, REHABILITATION, AND PROGNOSIS
WORKERS' COMPENSATION
MEDICAL REPORT

PREVENTION

The optimal strategy in dealing with occupational skin disease is its prevention. This is a multidisciplinary endeavor that requires planning by the employer, employee, government officials, and health care personnel to develop preventive measures. The responsibility for prevention of occupational skin disease rests on a number of individuals, including toxicologists, chemical and safety engineers, manufacturing management, industrial hygienists, workers, governmental regulators and scientists, and health care providers. It is the integration and cooperation among these various individuals that prevent occupational skin disease. There are multiple opportunities for intervention that can prevent occupational skin disease. These include identification of hazardous materials, identification of high-risk workers, and hazard control (Table 14-1).

> **It is the integration of hazardous chemical identification, preemployment screening, and hazard control by the employer, the worker, the government, and the health care profession that prevents occupational skin disease.**

Table 14-1	Prevention of Occupational Skin Disease

1. Hazardous material identification
2. Preemployment screening for identification of high-risk populations
3. Hazard control
    a. Employer measures
        (1) Engineering controls
        (2) Housekeeping
        (3) Warnings
        (4) Education and monitoring
    b. Worker
        (1) Personal protection
        (2) Hygiene
        (3) Education
    c. Government
        (1) Investigation
        (2) Regulations
        (3) Education
    d. Health care
        (1) Recognition of occupational dermatoses
        (2) Early therapy
        (3) Education

Hazardous Material Identification

The recognition of potentially hazardous chemicals should be accomplished by toxicologic testing before introduction into the workplace. For allergens and irritants, risk assessment testing can define the inherent irritant and allergenic properties of the chemical. This information may be found on the material safety data sheet and should be reviewed before new materials or processes are used. Questions can be elucidated by talking with the manufacturer of the raw material or industrial product. In addition, more information can be obtained by reviewing the cutaneous toxicity reported in the medical and toxicologic literature. Ideally, strong irritants and sensitizers will be identified before introduction into the workplace so that substitution with a less hazardous chemical can be accomplished or appropriate hazard control measures instituted. A number of chemicals that have caused occupational skin disease have been identified only after they have caused significant occupational skin disease in the workplace.

High-Risk Population Identification

Preemployment screening for the presence of selected skin diseases is helpful in identifying individuals who have a predisposition for work-related dermatoses or work aggravation of preexisting skin diseases. Workers should be questioned and examined for evidence of inflammatory diseases like atopic dermatitis and hand eczema so that these individuals can avoid jobs where there is significant exposure to irritants such as is found in health care workers and beauticians. Individuals with fair skin or sun sensitivity (i.e., lupus erythematosus) need to avoid occupations that have a significant amount of ultraviolet light exposure or use sunscreens. Individuals with psoriasis should avoid jobs in which recurrent friction and trauma are present, which because of the Koebner phenomenon, can cause exacerbation of their disease. If preemployment screening elicits a history suggestive of allergic contact dermatitis, preemployment patch testing may be recommended if the worker will have significant exposure to that allergen. Otherwise, preemployment patch testing is generally not recommended, since it has no predictive value concerning the future development of allergic contact dermatitis. Skin irritation tests with sodium hydroxide, dimethylsulfoxide, or sodium lauryl sulfate may be able to identify individuals at high risk for irritant contact dermatitis. However, the single test cannot be considered a valid screening. A much higher sensitivity can be achieved by applying a combination of irritancy tests.

It is critically important to carefully integrate the findings of preemployment health screening and job placement to achieve a balanced consideration of the employer's concerns while avoiding undue discrimination of the worker because of cutaneous disease. At minimum the preemployment screening identifies individuals who require specialized training in specific job assignments and closer medical observation.

> **Occupational exacerbation of preexisting skin disease can be avoided by preemployment screening of workers. However, overprotection with respect to job selection or restriction, even in high-risk disease groups, should be avoided.**

Hazard Control

Employer

The *employer* has several potential means of preventing occupational dermatoses, including environmental control, good housekeeping, warnings on hazardous material, and education of the workers. Ideally, exposure to hazardous chemicals can be eliminated by the engineering of closed systems that allow the manufacturing process to proceed without exposing the worker to harmful chemicals. Engineering systems such as automated samplers, computerized manufacturing, and robotic packaging may be implemented. Although this protects the line worker, consideration must also be given to maintenance personnel who may have exposure to hazardous chemicals. The goal of these engineering controls is to minimize cutaneous contamination. Environmental hygiene in the form of good housekeeping is indispensable in reducing worker exposure to irritants and allergens. Contaminated work surfaces from splattering, dripping, and spills can result in inadvertent skin contact. Housekeeping personnel responsible for environmental hygiene obviously must use appropriate industrial cleansers and wear appropriate protective clothing to prevent contact dermatitis. If skin exposure is from airborne contaminants, good ventilation for the removal of fumes, powders, dust, and aerosols is necessary. Ambient conditions such as heat and humidity are also important in avoiding such conditions as miliaria (heat rash), intertrigo, and xerotic (dry skin) eczema. Not only should material safety data sheets be available for worker perusal, but also, clearly written warning labels should be posted on hazardous materials. Education of supervisors and other management personnel should be accomplished, along with worker education. Appropriate prevention of occupational skin disease requires informed management and an informed worker. In addition, monitoring of occupational skin disease by the employer is helpful in identifying specific jobs and chemicals in a manufacturing process that are particularly hazardous to the worker.

Worker

The *worker* is critical in hazard control, since total avoidance of cutaneous contact with hazardous materials in many occupations cannot be accomplished by engineering controls alone. This requires the worker to use personal protection. Various types of protective clothing, such as gloves, aprons, sleeves, shoes, boots, and face shields, are available in a variety of materials like cloth, rubber, plastic, and metals. The protective clothing must fulfill requirements dictated by the type of physical and chemical exposure and the type of work being performed. The manufacturers of protective clothing can provide guidance for the appropriate selection of protective garments.

> **The employee and employer are both responsible for preventing occupational skin disease and must work together to achieve proper hazard control.**

Gloves. Because hand dermatitis is the most common site of occupational contact dermatitis, gloves are the most often used protective gear. Because a large number of gloves are available, knowledge of the physical and chemical properties of the glove; the potential severity of exposure to chemical, physical, and biologic hazards; and the job that is to be performed is required. Leather and textile gloves are used to prevent irritation from solids and reduce mechanical friction from dry materials. They can also protect against physical elements like cold and heat. In industries such as poultry processing, metal gloves prevent cuts and lacerations from knives and bones. In general, however, we use rubber or plastic gloves in the workplace to provide protection against chemical and biologic substances. The most common rubber glove materials are modified natural rubber: butyl, nitrile, chloroprene, styrene-butadiene, and fluoroelastomer. Plastic gloves are made from polyvinylchloride, polyethylene, polyvinyl alcohol, ethylene-methylmethacrylate, and polyurethane. Gloves can be manufactured from single, layered, or a mixture of materials.

Degradation and *permeation* are two types of chemical resistance properties that should be considered in the selection of gloves. The deterioration of the glove's physical properties, or degradation, can cause the glove to crack, tear easily, or dissolve so that large amounts of hazardous material come in contact with the skin. Once it is determined that the glove is not degraded by a hazardous chemical, the second consideration is how much of the chemical diffuses through the glove, or permeation. This is measured in the testing laboratory by breakthrough time and the steady-state permeation rate. The most important measure is breakthrough time, the time required for the chemical to be transported through the glove and detected by a testing device. For example, methyl methacrylate, the adhesive used for artificial orthopedic joints, readily penetrates through latex surgical gloves. Thus orthopedic surgeons have little protection from this hazardous material because the breakthrough time is so short. Although it is rarely done, the data for selecting a protective glove should be derived from testing under use conditions against workplace chemicals. Practical guidelines for the selection of gloves are available from the glove manufacturers, guidebooks, and databases (Tables 14-2, 14-3, and 14-4).

No single glove is protective from all possible chemicals.

It should be remembered that all glove materials are to some extent permeable to chemicals and that there is no universal protective material suitable for all possible chemicals. For some chemicals and some jobs there is no glove that gives a significant amount of protection. More harm than good can occur when chemicals permeate or spill into the glove and are trapped. Their harmful effect is exaggerated by occlusion, humidity, and skin temperature. Occasionally an allergy to a component of the glove or irritation from the glove itself can be the cause of contact dermatitis, not the hazardous chemical for which glove protection was intended. The gloves should not put the worker in jeopardy for getting caught in moving parts of machinery.

Workers with prolonged hand dermatitis should be referred for dermatologic examination and patch testing to rule out glove allergy. Gloves should fit well and not cause irritation themselves. Gauntlets should be long enough or gloves cuffed to prevent hazardous materials from getting inside. The gloves should be strong enough to resist cuts or punctures but at the same time provide enough dexterity to easily accomplish the job. Flocked or separately worn textile gloves under polymer gloves can prevent irritation and maceration from sweating. Extra gloves must be readily available to encourage workers to discard damaged or contaminated gloves. For the gloves to be effective, the worker must wear them conscientiously.

Table 14-2	Industrial Glove Manufacturers Who Provide Technical Support
Best Manufacturing Company Edison St. Menlo, GA 30731 Telephone: (800) 241-0323	North Hand Protection A Division of Siebe North, Inc. 4090 Azalea Dr. P.O. Box 70729 Charleston, SC 29415 Telephone: (803) 745-5900
Comasec Inc. P.O. Box 1219 8 Niblick Road Enfield, CN 06082 Telephone: (800) 333-0219	Pioneer Industrial Products 512 East Tiffin St. Willard, OH 44890 Telephone: (800) 537-2897
MSA RIDC Industrial Park 121 Gamma Dr. P.O. Box 426 Pittsburgh, PA 15238 Telephone: (412) 967-3000	MAPA Professional 512 East Tiffin St. Willard, OH 44890 Telephone: (800) 537-3897

> **Occupational skin disease has a guarded prognosis:**
> 1. **Twenty-five percent of cases clear.**
> 2. **Fifty percent improve.**
> 3. **Twenty-five percent are the same or worse.**

complete clearing; 50% improve but have periodic occurrences of the dermatitis; and 25% develop persistent dermatitis as severe or worse than the original condition. Factors that improve the prognosis include proper treatment and advice, retraining, and removal of the causative agent.

BIBLIOGRAPHY

Burrows D: Prognosis and factors influencing prognosis in industrial dermatitis, *Br J Dermatol* 105:65-70, 1981.

Cooley JE, Nethercott JR: Prognosis of occupational skin disease, *Occup Med* 9:19-24, 1994.

Hogan DJ, Dannaker CJ, Maibach HI: The prognosis of contact dermatitis, *J Am Acad Dermatol* 23:300-307, 1990.

Krutmann J, Morita A: Mechanisms of ultraviolet (UV) B and UVA phototherapy, *J Investig Dermatol Symp Proc* 4:70-72, 1999.

Lachapelle JM: Principles of prevention and protection in contact dermatitis (with special reference to occupational dermatology). In Rycroft RJG, Mennè T, Forsch PJ, editors: *Textbook of contact dermatitis,* New York, 1995, Springer-Verlag.

Nethercott JR, Holness DL: Follow-up study of workers with occupational contact dermatitis, *Contact Dermatitis* 23:241, 1990.

The National Institute for Occupational Safety and Health: Leading work-related diseases and injuries, *MMWR* 35:561-563, 1986.

WORKERS' COMPENSATION

Workers' compensation laws were an important development of the industrial revolution. They provided a satisfactory means of handling occupational disabilities as the economy evolved from being predominantly agricultural to industrial. These laws were first enacted in Germany in 1884, followed by Great Britain in 1897, the United States in 1911, and Canada in 1915. Before workers' compensation laws, the employee or the survivor, according to common law principle, sued the employer for damages that were due to employer negligence. This was a slow, costly, uncertain legal process that put the employee at a great disadvantage. Thus the essence of the workers' compensation laws that were enacted entitled the employee to medical treatment and compensation without regard to any fault and held that the employer should assume the cost of occupational disabilities. The workers' compensation statutes vary from country to country and from state to state within the United States. Various individuals become involved with these laws: the employer, the employee, insurance agents, attorneys, physicians, and administrators of the law. Workers' compensation laws should meet the following objectives:

1. Regardless of fault, provide occupationally induced illness or accident victims with a sure, prompt, reasonable income and medical benefits.
2. Reduce lengthy and costly court action.

3. Relieve public and private financial drains, since workers' compensation is paid for by the employer.
4. Encourage employer interest in safety and rehabilitation of the worker.
5. Promote investigation of the causes of accidents and disease, which will, it is hoped, reduce preventable human suffering.

Not all workers are covered by workers' compensation laws. For example, farm workers, domestic workers, and part-time employees usually do not have workers' compensation. A principal element of workers' compensation is to show that the injury or illness has an occupational causation and, in addition, to determine to what extent and for how long the worker is disabled.

> **Workers' compensation provides prompt medical and economic benefits to the employee in lieu of lengthy litigation to establish employer fault.**

The physician plays an important role in workers' compensation. This includes (1) providing care for the injured or diseased worker; (2) evaluating the relationship to work; (3) determining the degree and the period of disability; and (4) providing advice to the worker and industry about rehabilitation and preventive measures. It is critical that the physician weigh all these matters carefully, since the economic and social well-being of the worker depends on all these parameters, not just on the provision of good medical care. The authors have found that the physician's evaluation of the causal relationship, degree of disability, and advice to the worker and industry is often overlooked or poorly done because of ignorance or lack of physician time. Adequate evaluation of the worker requires an extended office visit to obtain a detailed occupational history as outlined in Chapter 13. If this is done, dealing with workers' compensation becomes relatively straightforward for the physician.

Establishing a causal relationship between work and skin conditions (90% being contact dermatitis) is one of the areas that seems to cause the most difficulty for the physician. Mathias (1989) very clearly outlined the criteria for establishing occupational causation and aggravation (Table 14-6). He suggested seven criteria that should be present before the clinician concludes that the dermatitis was occupationally induced. Any criterion that was answered negatively suggested that the dermatitis may not be work related. First, is the clinical appearance consistent with contact dermatitis? Other forms of dermatitis, like seborrheic dermatitis, atopic dermatitis, or dyshidrotic eczema may be present. A skin biopsy may be necessary to confirm the diagnosis of dermatitis. Second, are there cutaneous irritants or allergens in the workplace to which the worker is exposed? Are protective measures being taken? Third, does the occupational cutaneous exposure correlate with the distribution of dermatitis? Usually the areas of skin most severely affected are those with maximal exposure to the irritant or allergen. In most cases these are the hands or forearms. Fourth, is there a temporal relationship between exposure and the onset of dermatitis? The exposure must obviously precede the onset of contact dermatitis. Fifth, are nonoccupational causes excluded? For example, the dermatitis may be cannot be definitive in all these areas but requires follow-up visits and follow-up letters. Detail and accuracy are extremely important in the medical report, since it may have unintended repercussions. Before conclusions are made, it may be necessary to talk with the employee's supervisor and the manufacturers of chemicals found in the workplace.

Elements of the Medical Report
1. **Dermatologic history**
2. **Occupational history**
3. **Past dermatologic, medical, and social history**
4. **Skin examination**
5. **Patch test and laboratory results**
6. **Conclusions**
7. **Recommendations**

BIBLIOGRAPHY

Adams RM: Medicolegal aspects of occupational skin diseases, *Dermatol Clin* 6:121-129, 1988.

Burrows D, Donaldson AE: Preparing a medical report, *Clin Exper Dermatol* 19:206-209, 1994.

Emmett EA: The dermatologist and the right to know, *Dermatol Clin* 6:21-26, 1988.

Golstein A: Writing report letters for patients with skin disease resulting from on-the-job exposures, *Dermatol Clin* 2:631-641, 1984.

Himmelstein JS, Frumkin H: The right to know about toxic exposures: implications for physicians, *N Engl J Med* 312:687-690, 1985.

CHAPTER 15

Occupations Commonly Associated with Contact Dermatitis

AGRICULTURE WORKERS
CONSTRUCTION WORKERS
DENTAL WORKERS
ELECTRONICS WORKERS
FLORISTS
FOOD WORKERS
HAIRDRESSERS
HOUSEKEEPING PERSONNEL
MACHINISTS
MECHANICS
MEDICAL WORKERS
OFFICE WORKERS
PHOTOGRAPHERS
PRINTERS
TEXTILE WORKERS

In this chapter the occupations most commonly associated with contact dermatitis are discussed. It is important to understand the actual job performed by the occupational dermatology patient. This can be done vicariously in the office, but at some point a site visit may be necessary to gain full insight about the tasks performed by the worker, particularly when seeing a patient with an unfamiliar occupation. Some occupations, such as hairdressers, housekeeping personnel, nurses and physicians, dentists, dental assistants and dental hygienists, florists, and office workers, are found in all geographic locations and seen by every physician. Their jobs are familiar to us because we have made informal site visits when receiving their services. Other occupations are regionally distributed and are seen by some physicians but not others. It is necessary to become quite familiar with the workplace so that the evaluation of these workers becomes routine. In effect, the physician treating these workers becomes an expert in their industry's occupational dermatoses. It is important to establish good management and worker rapport to facilitate the evaluation, therapy, and prevention of occupational dermatitis.

> **The standard tray and supplemental allergens highlighted in the boxes for each occupation are the most important for patch testing.**

For each occupation in this chapter a brief description and the clinical aspects of the job are discussed. Although there are many similarities among workers doing the same job, individual differences make a detailed occupational history imperative. A suggested starting point for patch testing allergens is made. When all the patch test responses are negative, one should not feel totally confident that allergic contact dermatitis has been ruled out. The introduction of new materials into the workplace and the unavailability of some chemicals make it difficult to test with all workplace antigens. When possible, patch testing the actual materials from the workplace is the best means of avoiding false-negative results. At the same time, care must be taken to avoid false-positive irritant reactions, some of which may be severe. It is only with understanding the actual job duties, carefully evaluating the workplace materials, and correlating these with the eruption, that one can declare a case of dermatitis to be work related. A "halfway" investigation is inappropriate and often gets the physician, worker, and employer into trouble.

> **The investigation of occupational skin disease requires the following:**
> 1. **Understanding the job duties**
> 2. **Reviewing materials in the workplace**
> 3. **Patch testing with as many workplace materials as possible**
> 4. **Correlation of the eruption with the job**
> 5. **Establishing rapport with the employee and employer**

BIBLIOGRAPHY

Adams RM: Job descriptions with their irritants and allergens. In *Occupational skin disease,* ed 3, Philadelphia, 1999, WB Saunders.

Foussereau J, Benezra C, Maibach H: *Occupational contact dermatitis,* Philadelphia, 1982, WB Saunders.

Rietschel RL, Fowler JF: *Fisher's contact dermatitis,* ed 5, Baltimore, 2001, Williams & Wilkins.

Rycroft RJG, Mennè T, Frosch PJ, editors: *Textbook of contact dermatitis,* ed 2, New York, 1995, Springer-Verlag.

AGRICULTURE WORKERS
Job Description

Agriculture workers perform a variety of jobs and are exposed to a wide variety of chemical, biologic, and physical hazards. They grow crops that require preparing the soil for planting, as well as fertilizing, cultivating, and harvesting the crops (Figure 15-1). They raise and care for livestock: dairy cattle, beef, poultry, pigs, and sheep. They clean and repair farm equipment. They build and maintain fences and buildings. Farm workers are exposed to a number of different agricultural chemicals, veterinary medications, and feed additives. Environmental factors such as temperature, humidity, and frequent washing change the susceptibility of the skin to irritants and allergens. Farming has become so specialized that the occurrence of contact dermatitis very much depends on the type of farming done.

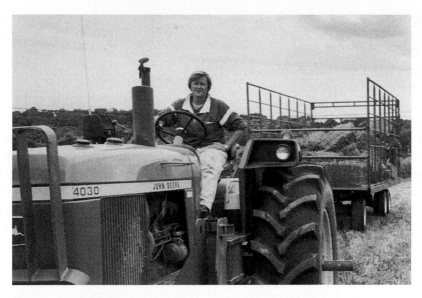

FIGURE 15-1
Farmer harvesting hay, which can cause irritant contact dermatitis.

Clinical Aspects

The United States had over 2 million farms in the mid-1980s that employed approximately 5 million workers. In California the agricultural sector had the highest rate of occupational skin disease, and agriculture had twice the rate of occupational skin disease as manufacturing. The risk and type of agricultural skin disease vary according to the crops, livestock, farming practices, and environs in which the farm is located. In California poison oak followed by pesticides was the leading cause of occupational skin disease in agricultural workers. Between 1990 and 1994 the Finnish Register of Occupational Diseases reported cow dander, disinfectants and detergents, wet and dirty work, and rubber chemicals to be the main causes of occupational hand eczema in farmers. Epidemiologic studies have shown that skin cancer is more common in farmers than in nonfarmers because of outdoor work and chronic ultraviolet light exposure. Farmers are also more likely to have skin infections from zoophilic agents such as *Trichophyton verrucosum,* the cause of superficial fungal infections.

Pesticides are used widely in agriculture to control insects, fungi, viruses, weeds, and rodents. In California alone, over 13,000 pesticide products that contain more than 800 active ingredients are registered. The highest rates of pesticide-related dermatitis in California have been in horticulture and crop services and are most often reported in field workers, especially in the grape industry. In addition to the active ingredients, inactive substances such as emulsifiers, surfactants, or biocides may cause irritation or allergic reactions. Skin exposure to pesticides occurs while mixing, loading, spraying, and cleaning equipment. Adequate skin protection is often lacking, particularly during very busy work periods and in hot weather. Washing facilities are generally not available in the field. The degree of skin contamination varies considerably with the degree of competent use and safety education. The U.S. Environmental Protection Agency has made recommendations to reduce worker exposure to pesticides that include (1) an adequate time interval between pesticide application and allowing workers into the field; (2) wearing of protective equipment such as gloves, aprons, footwear, and headgear when using pesticides; and (3) readily available decontamination provisions. Irritant reactions are commonly reported from contact with pesticides. Inorganic compounds, (e.g., copper sulfate) and fumigants (e.g., ethylene oxide, methyl bromide) are strongly irritating. Allergic reactions are apparently rare. When allergic contact dermatitis does occur, it is most likely from fungicides such as dithiocarbamates (maneb, carbofuran, carbaryl) and the thiophthalimides (captan, folpet, and captafol). A list of patch testing concentrations for pesticides and agricultural chemicals is provided by Hogan (1990).

Several feed additives (e.g., antibiotics, minerals, and antioxidants) have caused both irritant and allergic occupational contact dermatitis. These include furazolidone, tylosin, olaquindox, quindoxin, hydroquinone, halquinol, spiramycin, dinitromide, and virginiamycin.

Cultivated and wild plants have been a frequent cause of contact dermatitis among agriculture workers. As mentioned, poison oak and ivy are the most prominent causes of contact dermatitis. A report described a marked bullous dermatitis in field workers that was associated with exposure to the weed *Anthemis cotula* (mayweed). Phytophotodermatitis is well known after exposure to plants containing psoralens such as celery, wild parsnip, and cow parsley.

Animal materials, particularly cow dander in dairy farmers, may be one of the most important allergens in agriculturally induced skin disease. Immediate and delayed contact allergy to cow dander was a significant cause of hand eczema in Finnish dairy farmers. Some farmers had both immediate and delayed reactions; others had only one type of reaction; and others had positive contact urticaria only after a 20-minute patch test but not with prick tests.

Prevention

Agricultural workers are exposed to a multitude of natural and synthetic materials depending on the job they perform and crop or livestock raised. A detailed history provides clues to help direct patch testing. Identification and avoidance of putative irritants and allergens should help in ameliorating contact dermatitis.

Irritants and Allergens

Irritants
   Soaps and detergents
   Pesticides
   Dirt, moist dust, friction, sweating
   Disinfectants
   Solvents and petroleum products
   Fertilizers
   Plants and plant products
Allergens
   Standard tray
      Rubber chemicals (gloves, boots, hoses, pesticides)
      Potassium dichromate (leather, milk preservative, cement)

Preservatives (creams and ointments)
Sesquiterpene lactone mix (Compositae plants)
Supplemental trays
Pesticides (Trolab/Hermal)
Medicaments (Trolab/Hermal, Chemotechnique Diagnostics AB), feed
additives, veterinary drugs
Antimicrobials, preservatives (Trolab/Hermal): Disinfectants
Miscellaneous
Cow dander
Animal and plant materials
Flours, grains (fodder)
Storage mites, molds

> **The leading causes of dermatitis in farm workers are as follows:**
> **1. Poison oak/ivy**
> **2. Pesticides**

BIBLIOGRAPHY

Cellini A, Offidani A: An epidemiological study on cutaneous diseases of agricultural workers authorized to use pesticides, *Dermatology* 189:129-132, 1994.

de Groot AC, Conemans JM: Contact allergy to furazolidone, *Contact Dermatitis* 22:202-205, 1990.

Dinis A, Brandao M, Faria A: Occupational contact dermatitis from vitamin K_3 sodium bisulphite, *Contact Dermatitis* 18:170-171, 1988.

Hogan DJ: Pesticides and other agricultural chemicals. In Adams RM: *Occupational skin disease,* ed 2, Philadelphia, 1990, WB Saunders.

Lisi P, Caraffini S, Assalve D: Irritation and sensitization potential of pesticides, *Contact Dermatitis* 17:212-218, 1987.

Marks JG, Rainey CM, Rainey MA et al: Dermatoses among poultry workers: "chicken poison disease," *J Am Acad Dermatol* 9:852-857, 1983.

Mehler LN, O'Malley MA, Krieger RI: Acute pesticide morbidity and mortality: California, *Rev Environ Contam Toxicol* 129:51-66, 1992.

Neldner KH: Contact dermatitis from animal feed additives, *Arch Dermatol* 106:722-723, 1972.

O'Malley MA, Barba R: Bullous dermatitis in field workers associated with exposure to mayweed, *Am J Contact Dermat* 1:34-42, 1990.

Peachy RDG: Skin hazards in farming, *Br J Dermatol* 21:45-50, 1981.

Pentel MT, Andreozzi RJ, Marks JG: Allergic contact dermatitis from the herbicides trifluralin and benefin, *J Am Acad Dermatol* 31:1057-1058, 1994.

Sharma VK, Kaur S: Contact sensitization by pesticides in farmers, *Contact Dermatitis* 23:77-80, 1990.

Susitaival P, Hannuksela M: The 12-year prognosis of hand dermatosis in 896 Finnish farmers, *Contact Dermatitis* 32:233-237, 1995.

Susitaival P, Husman L, Hollmen A et al: Hand eczema in Finnish farmers: a questionnaire-based clinical study, *Contact Dermatitis* 32:150-155, 1995.

van Ginkel CJW, Sabapathy NN: Allergic contact dermatitis from the newly introduced fungicide fluazinam, *Contact Dermatitis* 32:160-162, 1995.

Veien NK: Hand eczema in farmers. In Mennè T, Maibach HI, editors: *Hand eczema,* Boca Raton, Fla, 1994, CRC.

CONSTRUCTION WORKERS

Job Description

Construction workers participate in a number of projects such as building houses, factories, schools, and hospitals. The construction industry employs a number of different workers, including carpenters, masons (Figure 15-2), electricians, painters, and plumbers. On some construction sites the same workers do all these tasks, and on others there is a division of labor.

Clinical Aspects

Carpenters do rough and finished woodworking such as framing houses, building concrete forms, and installing doors, windows, and molding. The nontropical woods (e.g., white pine) used by carpenters rarely cause allergic contact dermatitis. Wood preservatives have been reported to cause phototoxic reactions (creosote), chloracne (pentachlorophenol), and contact dermatitis (organic mecurials).

Masons and *cement workers* are at the greatest risk for allergic contact dermatitis in the construction industry. This is due to water-soluble hexavalent chromate in wet cement. Allergic contact dermatitis resulting from chromate is a ma-

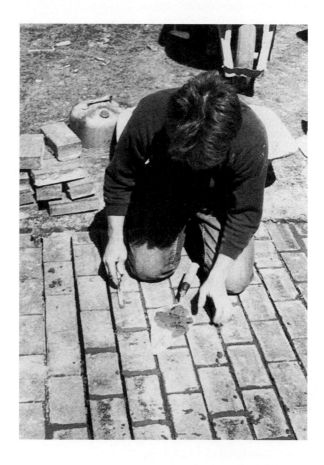

FIGURE 15-2
Mason laying a brick walk with cement that contains the allergen water-soluble hexavalent chromate. Cement is also an irritant.

jor cause of worker impairment and disability, particularly in workers who manufacture prefabricated concrete building units. In a recent German study, chromate was the main occupational allergen in construction workers, accounting for 44% patch test positivity of male construction workers compared with 4% in the male population without a construction background. The chromate content of cement varies significantly, depending on its source. Samples from European countries had ranges of 32 to 176 ppm of chromate, whereas samples of American cement revealed a chromate content from 5 to 124 ppm. Wet cement is also an irritant that can cause third-degree burns if allowed to have prolonged contact with the skin.

Electricians wire buildings and install various electrical fixtures such as lights. They use soldering fluxes that contain colophony to join wires together.

Painters cover holes and cracks with fillers and sand surfaces before painting. Paints are composed of pigments, binding materials, solvents, and biocides if water based. The binding materials are natural oils and gums or synthetic resins. Turpentine is one of the most common sensitizers in painters, with the geographic source of the turpentine determining its allergenicity. For example, French turpentine is much less allergenic than Scandinavian turpentine. Synthetic resin paints contain the allergens formaldehyde, epoxy, and acrylic compounds. Water-based latex paints contain a number of different biocides, particularly the isothiazolinones, that may cause allergic contact dermatitis.

Plumbers cut, fit, and install metal and plastic pipes that carry liquids or gases. They are exposed to irritant cleansers, adhesives, and soldering fluxes that contain colophony.

Irritants and Allergens

Irritants
    Cleansers and solvents
    Dirt and refuse
    Wet cement
    Fiberglass
    Resins
Allergens
    Standard tray
        Potassium dichromate (cement, leather gloves and boots, wood
           preservative)
        Rubber chemicals (gloves, tool handles, electrical wiring, boots)
        Epoxy resin (paints and adhesives)
        Colophony (soldering flux, coating on nails, pine dust)
        p-tert-Butylphenol formaldehyde resin (adhesives)
        Nickel sulfate (hand tools)
        Formaldehyde (phenolic resins, metal cleaners)
    Supplemental trays
        Antimicrobials, preservatives (Trolab/Hermal): Biocides used in paints
        Plastics, glues, epoxy (Trolab/Hermal, Chemotechnique Diagnostics AB):
           Resins found in paints and adhesives
    Additional allergens: Turpentine (solvent)

> **The most frequent allergen for construction workers is water-soluble hexavalent chromate in cement.**

BIBLIOGRAPHY

Avnstorp C: Cement eczema. In Mennè T, Maibach HI, editors: *Exogenous dermatoses: environmental dermatitis,* Boca Raton, Fla, 1991, CRC.

Condè-Salazar L, Guimaraens D, Villegas C et al: Occupational allergic contact dermatitis in construction workers, *Contact Dermatitis* 33:226-230, 1995.

Correia O, Barros MA, Mesquita-Guimaraes J: Airborne contact dermatitis from the woods *Acacia melanoxylon* and *Entandophragma cylindricum, Contact Dermatitis* 27:343-344, 1992.

Fischer T, Bohlin S, Edling C et al: Skin disease and contact sensitivity in house painters using water-based paints, glues, and putties, *Contact Dermatitis* 32:39-45, 1995.

Fregert S: Chromium valencies and cement dermatitis, *Br J Dermatol* 105:7-9, 1981.

Fregert S: Construction work. In Maibach HI, editor: *Occupational and industrial dermatology,* ed 2, Chicago, 1987, Year Book Medical.

Gebhardt M: Construction workers. In Gebhardt M, Elsner P, Marks JG, editors: *Handbook of contact dermatitis,* London, 2000, Martin Dunitz.

Geier J, Schnuch A: Kontaktallergien im Bauhauptgewerbe, *Dermatosen* 36:109-114, 1998.

Goh CL: Hand eczema in the construction industry. In Mennè T, Maibach HI, editors: *Hand eczema,* Boca Raton, Fla, 1994, CRC.

Goh CL, Gan SL, Ngui SJ: Occupational dermatitis in a prefabrication construction factory, *Contact Dermatitis* 15:235-240, 1986.

Kiec-Swierczynska M: Occupational dermatoses and allergy to metals in Polish construction workers manufacturing prefabricated building units, *Contact Dermatitis* 23:27-32, 1990.

Mackey SA, Marks JG: Allergic contact dermatitis to white pine sawdust, *Arch Dermatol* 128:1660, 1992.

Moura C, Dias M, Vale T: Contact dermatitis in painters, polishers and varnishers, *Contact Dermatitis* 31:51-53, 1994.

DENTAL WORKERS

Job Description

Dentists fill, extract, straighten, and replace teeth and perform oral surgical procedures. Dental hygienists clean, x-ray, and examine teeth. Dental assistants help the dentist in performing procedures, take and develop x-ray films, and make amalgams, composite resins, and impression material (Figure 15-3). The dental laboratory technician fabricates and repairs dental prostheses.

Clinical Aspects

Hand dermatitis in dental workers is common with frequencies reported from 20% to 40%. Recent questionnaire studies in Denmark revealed a 1-year prevalence of occupationally related dermatitis in dentists (21.4%) and in dental technicians (43%). Frequent hand washing by dental personnel results in drying and chapping of the hands, which causes irritant contact dermatitis. In a German study, the skin disease of 24% of dental technicians with suspected occupational contact dermatitis had an irritant cause. In addition to wet work, grinding and physical irritation caused by polishing metals and plastic materials were identified as causative agents. Other common contact irritants in dental occupations are soaps, detergents, and disinfectants.

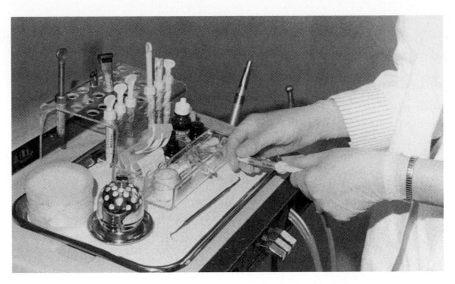

FIGURE 15-3
Dental assistant preparing composite resin, which contains sensitizing epoxy and acrylate compounds.

The use of biocides, particularly those containing glutaraldehyde for cold sterilization of instruments and disinfection of countertops, is a frequent cause of allergic contact dermatitis in dentists, hygienists, and assistants. Chlorine dioxide solutions (Exspor) can be substituted for glutaraldehyde for immersion sterilization of patient treatment items that cannot be heat sterilized.

Allergic and irritant contact dermatitis and contact urticaria from latex gloves are more frequent in dental personnel, since they began wearing gloves to prevent infections with the herpes simplex and human immunodeficiency viruses.

The local anesthetic procaine was once a significant cause of allergic contact dermatitis in dentists. With the introduction of lidocaine, which has a low sensitizing potential, allergy to local anesthetics has been almost totally eliminated.

Monofunctional acrylics such as methyl methacrylate and 2-hydroxyethyl methacrylate, polyfunctional acrylics such as ethylene glycol dimethacrylate and triethylene glycol diacrylate, and acrylated and methacrylated prepolymer such as bis-GMA or urethane dimethacrylate are important sensitizing compounds in the dental profession. Dental composite resin products based on bisphenol A and (meth) acrylates that are used for restorations and dentures have become a prominent cause of allergic contact dermatitis in dental personnel. They contain several sensitizers, including (1) prepolymers, which are usually acrylated epoxies or acrylated urethanes; and (2) monofunctional or multifunctional aliphatic (meth) acrylates and additives that include initiators (benzoyl peroxide), activators (tertiary aromatic amines), and inhibitors (hydroquinone). The catalysts from the two impression materials Impregum and Scutum, which are used for crowns, have also caused allergic contact dermatitis.

Mercury and metals (aluminum, copper, gold, palladium, platinum, silver, and tin) in modern alloys seem to be an uncommon cause of allergic contact dermatitis today.

Prevention

Protective gloves and "no-touch" techniques should be used to prevent irritant and allergic contact dermatitis in dental workers.

Irritants and Allergens

Irritants
 Frequent hand washing
 Gloves
 Antiseptics
 Soaps, detergents
 Physical irritation (polishing dusts, grinding)
Allergens
 Standard tray
  Rubber chemicals (gloves)
  Epoxy (dental composite resin)
 Supplemental trays
  Dental (Trolab/Hermal, Chemotechnique Diagnostics AB): Mercury
   (amalgam)
   Methylmethacrylate (dental prostheses)
   Eugenol (analgesic)
   Bis-GMA (dental composite resin)
 Antimicrobials preservatives (Trolab/Hermal): Glutaraldehyde (disinfectant)
 Additional allergens: Dental composite resin, 1% in petrolatum

> **The most common dental allergens are:**
> 1. **Glutaraldehyde**
> 2. **Rubber chemicals**
> 3. **Composite resins**

BIBLIOGRAPHY

Farli M, Gasperini M, Francalanci S et al: Occupational contact dermatitis in two dental technicians, *Contact Dermatitis* 22:282-287, 1990.

Field EA: The use of powdered gloves in dental practice: a cause to concern? *J Dent* 25:209-214, 1997.

Kanerva L, Estlander T, Jolanki R: Allergic contact dermatitis from dental composite resins due to aromatic epoxy acrylates and aliphatic acrylates, *Contact Dermatitis* 20:201-211, 1989.

Kanerva L, Estlander T, Jolanki R: Occupational skin allergy in the dental profession, *Dermatol Clin* 12:517-532, 1994.

Kanerva L, Estlander T, Jolanki R: Allergy caused by acrylics: past, present, and prevention, *Prev Contact Dermatitis* 25:86-96, 1996.

Kanerva L, Henrikseckerman ML, Estlander T, Jolanki R: Dentist's occupational allergic paronychia and contact dermatitis caused by acrylics, *Eur J Dermatol* 7:177-180, 1997.

Kanerva L, Turjanmaa K, Estlander T et al: Occupational allergic contact dermatitis caused by 2-hydroxyethyl methacrylate (2-HEMA) in a new dentin adhesive, *Am J Contact Dermat* 2:24-30, 1991.

Munksgaard EC, Hansen EK, Engen T, Holm U: Selfreported occupational dermatological reactions among Danish dentists, *Eur J Oral Sci* 104:396-402, 1996.

Mürer AJ, Poulsen OM, Roed-Petersen J, Tüchsen F: Skin problems among Danish dental technicians, *Contact Dermatitis* 33:42-47, 1995.

Rustemeyer T, Frosch PJ: Occupational skin disease in dental laboratory technicians (I). Clinical picture and causative factors, *Contact Dermatitis* 34:125-133, 1996.

Uveges RE, Grimwood RE, Slawsky LD, Marks JG: Epidemiology of hand dermatitis in dental personnel, *Military Med* 160:335-338, 1995.

ELECTRONICS WORKERS

Job Description

The electronics industry is a large, diverse, worldwide conglomerate. In the United States it is the largest employer in the manufacturing sector and makes commercial, consumer, and military products. The major processes in the electronics industry are the fabrication and assembly of semiconductors, printed circuit boards, and the final product. This requires a number of individual steps including wafer preparation, soldering, electroplating, printing, etching, glass-blowing, cutting, drilling, testing, and packaging. Evaluating the electronics worker requires understanding the specific job performed.

Clinical Aspects

Despite the widespread use of chemicals in the electronics industry, irritant and allergic contact dermatitis is relatively infrequent. This is probably due in large part to closed systems that result in reduced worker contact with these chemicals. The most common and notorious irritant chemical in the semiconductor industry is hydrofluoric acid, which is used in wafer etching and polishing. It is reputed to be the most common cause of burns. Irritant contact dermatitis has also been reported from soldering fluxes, solvents, etching chemicals, and cleaning agents.

Soldering (Figure 15-4) is a common procedure in which two metals are joined together by using solder as the filler metal. Flux is used to clean the metal surfaces to be joined and allow the solder to flow smoothly to form a good joint. Soldering fluxes contain irritating acids and solvents and the allergens colophony, aminoethylethanolamine, and hydrazine. The type of flux varies, depending on the type of soldering work required. In the assembly of printed circuit boards, aminoethylethanolamine-based fluxes are more common than colophony- and hydrazine-containing fluxes. Typically the dermatitis from soldering fluxes begins on the fingers periungually and then may spread to involve the dorsum of the hands and forearms. The majority of workers have irritant contact dermatitis from fluxes, but some have allergic contact dermatitis. The use of cotton gloves exacerbates the condition, since the gloves tend to become soaked with the flux, thus resulting in prolonged skin contact. Workers who minimize flux contact by wearing plastic or rubber gloves or finger cots appear to have a good prognosis.

Epoxy and acrylate resins are used for die attachment, device encapsulation, ingot mounting, photoresists, and anaerobic sealants, among other functions. The resins and their hardeners are well-known irritants and allergens causing contact dermatitis of the hands and airborne allergic contact dermatitis of exposed skin.

Metals are another cause of allergic contact dermatitis among electronic workers. Potassium and sodium dichromate solutions are used in wafer cutting and etching. The workers are also exposed to gold in electroplating, cobalt from magnet manufacturing, nickel in alloys and tools, and platinum that is used for connections.

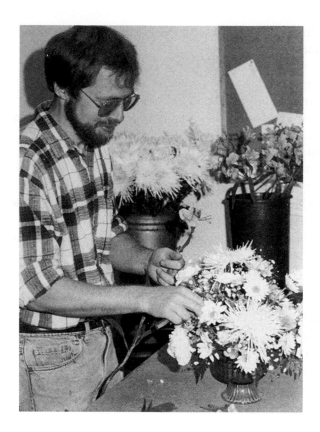

FIGURE 15-5
Designer/arranger making a floral display with *Alstroemeria* species and chrysanthemums, which can cause allergic contact dermatitis.

Clinical Aspects

Exposure to soaps, detergents, water, fertilizers, pesticides, and irritating plants has been linked to dermatitis in floral workers. In a North American survey, at least one third of retail florist shops reported an employee with skin problems. Hausen and Oestmann (1988) found approximately every other florist and gardener with skin disease to be allergic to plants. Concern about the increasing incidence of hand dermatitis in floral shop workers in the United States prompted Thiboutot and others (1990) to investigate the prevalence and cause of hand dermatitis at a large floral company. Twenty-six percent of the workers reported hand dermatitis within the previous 12 months. Patch testing to the standard, perfume, pesticide, and plant trays revealed that the most frequent positive patch test reaction was to tuliposide A, the allergen in *Alstroemeria* species (see Chapter 10). Florists allergic to *Alstroemeria* species also need to avoid tulips, since tuliposide A is also found in the stem, leaf, petal, and bulbs of tulips.

Chrysanthemum is the other plant that frequently causes allergic contact dermatitis in florists. The two most common species are *Chrysanthemum morifolium* and *Chrysanthemum indicum* (see Chapter 10). Because the chrysanthemum is a member of the Compositae family of plants, the allergens in chrysanthemums are sesquiterpene lactones, including alantolactone, parthenolide, and arteglasin A. No single sesquiterpene lactone or the sesquiterpene lactone mix (see Chapter 5) is adequate to screen for chrysanthemum allergy. It is recommended that portions of the specific chrysanthemum plant handled by the florist be tested.

Another allergenic plant that may be handled by florists is the English primrose, *Primula obconica* (see Chapter 10). This is a popular household plant that also causes dermatitis in housewives. Patch testing is best done with synthetic primin (see Chapter 5) rather than with parts of the plant.

There are dozens of other potential substances that may cause allergic contact dermatitis, including pesticides, fragrances, and preservatives. These, however, seem to be infrequent allergens in florists.

Although sensitization seems to be a predominant irritant cause of contact dermatitis in florists, cumulative irritation due to repeated wet work and minor trauma from items such as thorns, stems, wires, and irritant sap from plants can also lead to skin problems. *Narcissus, Dieffenbachia* (dumb cane), and *Euphorbia* (spurge) are examples of potent irritant plants.

Prevention

Prevention of allergic contact dermatitis due to *Alstroemeria* species requires avoidance of the plant or the wearing of latex nitrile gloves. Vinyl gloves are ineffective in preventing the penetration of tuliposide A. Many florists are either unable or unwilling to wear gloves. Avoidance of chrysanthemums is much more difficult, since this cut flower is universally used in floral arrangements.

Irritants and Allergens

Irritants
    Wet work
    Microtrauma (tools, stems, thorns, wire)
    Plants
Allergens
    Standard tray
        Nickel (tools)
        Rubber chemicals (gloves)
        Fragrance mix (fragrances)
        Balsam of Peru (fragrances)
        Primin *(Primula obconica)*
        Sesquiterpene lactone mix (chrysanthemum)
    Supplemental trays
        Pesticides (Trolab/Hermal)
        Fragrances (Trolab/Hermal, Chemotechnique Diagnostics AB)
    Additional allergens
        Tuliposide A, α-methylene-γ-butyrolactone, or portions of *Alstroemeria*
            plant (stem, petal, and leaf)
        Portions of chrysanthemum (stem, petal, leaf)

The most frequent allergens in florists are:
1. **Tuliposide A (*Alstroemeria* species)**
2. **Sesquiterpene lactones (chrysanthemum)**

BIBLIOGRAPHY

Bangha E, Elsner P: Occupational contact dermatitis towards sesquiterpene lactones in a florist, *Am J Contact Dermat* 7:188-190, 1996.

Crippa M, Misquith L, Lonati A et al: Dyshidrotic eczema and sensitization to dithiocarbamates in a florist, *Contact Dermatitis* 23:203-204, 1990.

Gette MT, Marks JG: Tulip fingers, *Arch Dermatol* 126:203-205, 1990.

Ippen I, Wereta-Kubek M, Rose U: Haut-und Schleimhautreaktionen durch Zimmerpflanzen der Gattung Dieffenbachia, *Derm Beruf Umwelt* 34:93-101, 1986.

Julian CG, Bowers PW: The nature and distribution of daffodil pickers' rash, *Contact Dermatitis* 37:259-262, 1997.

Marks JG: Allergic contact dermatitis to *Alstroemeria, Arch Dermatol* 124:914-916, 1988.

Merrick C, Fenney J, Clarke EC et al: A survey of skin problems in floristry, *Contact Dermatitis* 24:306, 1991.

Santucci B, Picardo M: Occupational contact dermatitis to plants, *Clin Dermatol* 10:157-165, 1992.

Schmidt RJ, Kingston T: Chrysanthemum dermatitis in South Wales: diagnosis by patch testing with feverfew (*Tanacetum parthenium* extract), *Contact Dermatitis* 13:120-121, 1985.

Thiboutot DM, Hamory BH, Marks JG: Dermatoses among floral shop workers, *J Am Acad Dermatol* 22:54-58, 1990.

Ueda A, Aoyama K, Manda F et al: Delayed-type allergenicity of triforine (Saprol), *Contact Dermatitis* 31:140-145, 1994.

Urishibata O, Kase K: Irritant contact dermatitis from *Euphorbia marginata, Contact Dermatitis* 24:155-156, 1991.

FOOD WORKERS

Job Description

Food workers clean (Figure 15-6), prepare, and cook a number of gastronomic items, including fruits, vegetables, spices, dairy products, fish, meats, poultry, and baked goods. Occupational exposure to different foods varies depending on the specific job, such as caterer, chef, short-order cook, housekeeper, delicatessen worker, bartender, green grocer, butcher, or baker. The evaluation of food workers obviously must be tailored to the foods that they handle.

Clinical Aspects

Irritant contact dermatitis, allergic contact dermatitis, and contact urticaria are the most frequent skin reactions from handling foods. Irritant contact dermatitis is due to wet work, irritating foods, and repeated exposure to soaps and detergents.

Allergic contact dermatitis has been reported from many foods. The main allergens, however, are garlic and onion. These two plants belong to the family Alliaceae. They are the most common cause of dermatitis in caterers and housewives, which is manifested as a dry, fissured, hyperkeratotic eczema of the fingertips. The allergens in garlic are diallyldisulfide and allicin. The allergen in onion has not been identified. Patch testing with cut raw onion and garlic should be done cautiously, since they are also irritants. Positive test results to the raw onion or garlic should be confirmed with a 10% aqueous extract of these vegetables or, for garlic, diallyldisulfide 1% in petrolatum.

Contact urticaria, as well as contact dermatitis, is produced by many foods

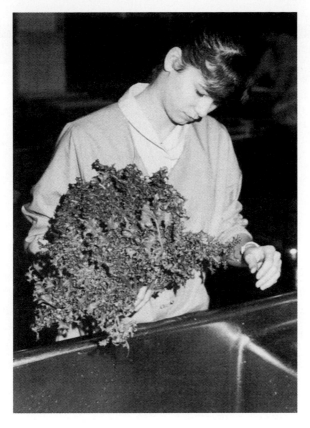

FIGURE 15-6
Food worker cleaning endive, which can cause irritant contact dermatitis from wet work or allergic contact dermatitis from sesquiterpene lactones in the endive.

(Table 15-1). Hjorth and Roed-Petersen (1976) described a type of contact urticaria that they called protein contact dermatitis. Rather than the classic wheal-and-flare reaction typical of urticaria, in the affected chefs and sandwich makers, swelling, itching, stinging, and vesiculation developed within minutes of contact with proteinaceous foods, particularly fish and shellfish.

Phototoxic reactions have occurred after handling lime and celery. These reactions are due to furocoumarins that are present within the plant. Other vegetables that contain furocoumarins include parsley, figs, and parsnips.

Bakers are exposed to flour, flour additives, flavors, and dyes. Flour may cause both immediate and delayed-type hypersensitivity reactions. Ammonium persulfate and benzoyl peroxide are used as flour bleaches. Ammonium persulfate has been banned as an additive in some countries because it can cause contact urticaria and occasionally severe anaphylactic reactions. A common flour additive, α-amylase, is used to facilitate rising of dough, improve flavor, and extend shelf-life. It causes contact urticaria and dermatitis in bakers with hand eczema. Flavors, particularly cinnamon, have caused allergic contact dermatitis in bakers. Food dyes rarely sensitize. Mechanization of bakeries has diminished irritant contact dermatitis to flour and dough. However, a recent German prospective

Table 15-1	Common Food Substances That May Cause Contact Urticaria and Contact Dermatitis						
Dairy Products	**Fish**	**Fruits**	**Grains**	**Hot Spices** **Meats**	**Nuts** **Vegetables**	**Vegetables— cont'd**	
Cheese	Cod	Apple	Flour	Beef	Beans	Lettuce	
Egg	Mackerel	Banana	Malt	Chicken	Carrot	Onion	
Milk	Prawns	Orange	Wheat	Lamb	Celery	Parsnip	
	Shrimp	Peach		Liver	Cucumber	Potato	
		Plum		Turkey	Garlic	Rutabaga	
						Tomato	

From Mathias CGT: *Occup Health Safety* 53:53-56, 1984.

epidemiological cohort study in baker apprentices still revealed irritant hand dermatitis in 29% after 6 months of work.

Food additives such as preservatives, antioxidants, and emulsifiers have occasionally been reported to cause allergic contact dermatitis. Gallate esters (dodecyl, octyl, and propyl) used as antioxidants in foods and washing powder have caused occupational contact allergy. The antioxidants butylated hydroxyanisole (BHA) and butylated hydroxytoluene (BHT) have also rarely produced allergic contact dermatitis.

Prevention

Prevention of hand dermatitis in food workers can be a challenge. Avoiding irritating foods and reduced hand washing are necessary. Wearing gloves may be impractical, but gloves should be used if possible. Identifying the offending food and avoidance are the best solutions.

Irritants and Allergens

Irritants
  Wet work
  Soaps and detergents
  Fish, meat
  Spices
  Vegetable and fruit juices
  Garlic and onion
  Flour and dough
Allergens
  Standard tray
    Rubber chemicals (gloves)
    Balsam of Peru, cinnamic aldehyde, fragrance mix (flavors, spices)
    Metals (kitchen utensils)
    Sesquiterpene lactone mix (food plants [e.g., lettuce, endive, chicory, artichoke])
  Supplemental trays
    Perfumes, flavors (Trolab/Hermal): Essential oils used for flavoring
    Bakery (Chemotechnique Diagnostics AB): Food preservatives, flavors

Additional allergens
Food as is (confirm positive reactions with controls)
Diallyldisulfide (Chemotechnique Diagnostics AB): Garlic
Dipentene (Trolab/Hermal): Citrus fruits

> **Many foods cause both contact urticaria and allergic contact dermatitis. The most common causes of contact urticaria are:**
> **1. Fish**
> **2. Shellfish**
> **The most common causes of allergic contact dermatitis are:**
> **1. Garlic**
> **2. Onions**

BIBLIOGRAPHY

Acciai MC, Francalanci BS, Giorgini S, Sertoli A: Allergic contact dermatitis in caterers, *Contact Dermatitis* 28:48, 1993.

Audicana M, Bernaola G: Occupational contact dermatitis from citrus fruits: lemon essential oils, *Contact Dermatitis* 31:183-185, 1994.

Bauer A, Bartsch R, Stadeler M et al: Development of occupational skin diseases during vocational training in baker and confectioner apprentices: a follow-up study, *Contact Dermatitis* 39:307-311, 1998.

Camarasa J: Foods. In Guin JD, editor: *Practical contact dermatitis: a handbook for the practitioner,* New York, 1995, McGraw-Hill.

Chan EF, Mowad C: Contact dermatitis to foods and spices, *Am J Contact Dermat* 9:71-79, 1998.

Cronin E: Dermatitis of the hands in caterers, *Contact Dermatitis* 17:265-269, 1987.

de Groot AC, Gerkens F: Occupational airborne contact dermatitis from octyl gallate, *Contact Dermatitis* 23:184-205, 1990.

Halkier-Sorensen L, Heickendorff L, Dalsgaard I et al: Skin symptoms among workers in the fish processing industry are caused by high-molecular-weight compounds, *Contact Dermatitis* 24:94-100, 1991.

Hausen BM, Hjorth N: Skin reactions to topical food exposure, *Dermatol Clin* 2:567-578, 1984.

Hjorth N: Occupational dermatitis in the catering industry, *Br J Dermatol* 105:37-40, 1981.

Hjorth N, Roed-Petersen J: Occupational protein contact dermatitis in food handlers, *Contact Dermatitis* 2:28-42, 1976.

Krook G: Occupational dermatitis from *Lactuca sativa* (lettuce) and *Cichorium* (endive): simultaneous occurrence of immediate and delayed allergy as a cause of contact dermatitis, *Contact Dermatitis* 3:27-36, 1977.

Lembo G, Balato N, Patruno C et al: Allergic contact dermatitis due to garlic *(Allium sativum),* *Contact Dermatitis* 25:330-331, 1991.

Marks JG, Rainey CM, Rainey MA et al: Dermatoses among poultry workers: "chicken poison disease," *J Am Acad Dermatol* 9:852-857, 1983.

Mathias CGT: Food substances may cause skin reactions among handlers, *Occup Health Safety* 53:53-56, 1984.

McFadden JP, White IR, Rycroft RJG: Allergic contact dermatitis from garlic, *Contact Dermatitis* 27:333-334, 1992.

Morren MA, Janssens V, Dooms-Goossens A et al: α-Amylase, a flour additive: an important cause of protein contact dermatitis in bakers, *J Am Acad Dermatol* 29:723-728, 1993.

Nethercott JR, Holness DL: Occupational dermatitis in food handlers and bakers, *J Am Acad Dermatol* 21:485-490, 1989.

dermatitis occurs, it is important to reduce its severity and clear it as quickly as possible, to prevent self-perpetuation of an unmasked endogenous eczema despite the affected individual's leaving work.

Prevention

Prevention of contact dermatitis in hairdressers can be difficult. Reduced frequency or elimination of shampooing obviously helps the individual with irritant contact dermatitis. For hairdressers with allergies to *p*-phenylenediamine, wearing latex nitrile gloves appears to be helpful in preventing allergic contact dermatitis from permanent hair dyes. For those who are allergic to glyceryl thioglycolate, the usual gloves are not protective, and avoidance of acid permanent waves is mandatory. In contrast to permanent hair colors, which are nonantigenic after oxidation in dyed hair, glyceryl thioglycolate–related allergens in acid permanent waves remain in hair for months and can continue to cause allergic contact dermatitis in the hairdresser and the client. Therefore hairdressers who are allergic to glyceryl thioglycolate should avoid cutting a client's hair for a couple of months after acid permanent waves.

> **Prevention of hand dermatitis in hairdressers*:**
> 1. **Wash infrequently and use moisturizers**
> 2. **Wear disposable vinyl gloves for shampooing, bleaching, drying, and perms**
> 3. **Avoid nickel in all jewelry and tools**
> 4. **Keep workplace clean**
> *Modified from van der Walle HB: *Contact Dermatitis* 30:265-270, 1994.

Irritants and Allergens

Irritants
  Shampoos
  Permanent-wave solutions
  Wet work
  Hydrogen peroxide
  Ammonium persulfate
  Dry air
  Low-grade repetitive friction
  Gloves
Allergens
  Standard tray
    Nickel (tools such as scissors, clips)
    Rubber chemicals (gloves)
    Preservatives (cosmetics)
    p-Phenylenediamine (permanent hair dyes)
    Cinnamic aldehyde, fragrance mix, and Balsam of Peru (fragrances)
  Supplemental trays
    Hairdressing (Trolab/Hermal, Chemotechnique Diagnostics AB)
      Glyceryl thioglycolate (GTG) (acid permanent-waving solution)
      Ammonium persulfate (hair bleach)
    Fragrances (Trolab/Hermal, Chemotechnique Diagnostics AB)

The most frequent allergens in hairdressers are:
1. *p*-Phenylenediamine
2. Glyceryl thioglycolate
3. Nickel
4. Ammonium persulfate

BIBLIOGRAPHY

Bauer A: Hairdressers. In Gebhardt M, Elsner P, Marks JG, editors: *Handbook of contact dermatitis,* London, 2000, Martin Dunitz.

Calnan CD, Shuster S: Reactions to ammonium persulfate, *Arch Dermatol* 88:812-815, 1963.

Conde-Salazar L, Baz M, Guimaraens D, Cannavo A: Contact dermatitis in hairdressers: patch test results in 379 hairdressers (1980-1993), *Am J Contact Dermat* 6:19-23, 1995.

Cronin E: *Contact dermatitis,* New York, 1980, Churchill Livingstone.

Cronin E, Kullavanijaya P: Hand dermatitis in hairdressers, *Acta Derm Venereol (Stockh)* 85:47-50, 1979.

Frosch PJ, Burrows D, Camarasa JG et al: Allergic reactions to a hairdressers' series: results from 9 European centres, *Contact Dermatitis* 28:180-183, 1993.

Guerra L, Tosti A, Bardazzi F et al: Contact dermatitis in hairdressers: the Italian experience, *Contact Dermatitis* 26:101-107, 1992.

Hannuksela M, Hassi J: Hairdresser's hand, *Dermatosen* 28:149-151, 1980.

Holness DL, Nethercott JR: Epicutaneous testing results in hairdressers, *Am J Contact Dermat* 4:224-234, 1990.

James J, Calnan CD: Dermatitis of the hands in ladies' hairdressers, *J Trans St John's Hosp Dermatol Soc* 42:19-42, 1959.

Katsarou A, Koufou B, Takou K et al: Patch test results in hairdressers with contact dermatitis in Greece (1985-1994), *Contact Dermatitis* 33:347-361, 1995.

Kellett JK, Beck MH: Ammonium persulfate sensitivity in hairdressers, *Contact Dermatitis* 13:26-28, 1985.

Lynde CW, Mitchell JC: Patch test results in 66 hairdressers (1973-1981), *Contact Dermatitis* 8:302-307, 1982.

Marks JG: Occupational skin disease in hairdressers, *Occup Med* 1:273-284, 1986.

Marks R, Cronin E: Hand eczema in hairdressers, *Aust J Dermatol* 18:123-126, 1977.

Matsunaga K, Hosokawa K, Suzuki M et al: Occupational allergic contact dermatitis in beauticians, *Contact Dermatitis* 18:94-96, 1988.

Morrison LH, Storrs FJ: Persistence of an allergen in hair after glyceryl monothioglycolate–containing permanent wave solutions, *J Am Acad Dermatol* 19:52-59, 1988.

Pilz B, Frosch PJ: Hairdressers' eczema. In Menne T, Maibach HI, editors: *Hand eczema,* Boca Raton, Fla, 1994, CRC.

Storrs FJ: Permanent wave contact dermatitis: contact allergy to glyceryl monothioglycolate, *J Am Acad Dermatol* 11:74-85, 1984.

Sutthipisal N, McFadden JP, Cronin E: Sensization in atopic and nonatopic hairdressers with hand eczema, *Contact Dermatitis* 29:206-209, 1993.

van der Walle HB, Brunsveld VM: Dermatitis in hairdressers. I. The experience of the past 4 years, *Contact Dermatitis* 30:217-221, 1994.

van der Walle, HB: Dermatitis in hairdressers. II. Management and prevention, *Contact Dermatitis* 30:265-270, 1994.

van der Walle HB, Brunsveld VM: Latex allergy among hairdressers, *Contact Dermatitis* 32:177-178, 1995.

Wahlberg JE: Nickel allergy and atopy in hairdressers, *Contact Dermatitis* 1:161-165, 1975.

BIBLIOGRAPHY

Desciak EB, Marks JG: Dermatoses among housekeeping personnel, *Am J Contact Dermat* 8:32-34, 1997.

Flyvholm MA: Contact allergens in registered cleaning agents for industrial and household use, *Br J Indust Med* 50:1043-1050, 1993.

Foussereau J, Benezra C, Maibach HI: *Occupational contact dermatitis: clinical and chemical aspects,* Philadelphia, 1982, WB Saunders.

Hansen KS: Occupational dermatoses in hospital cleaning women, *Contact Dermatitis* 9:343-351, 1983.

Sussman GL, Lem D, Liss G, Beezhol D: Latex allergy in housekeeping personnel, *Ann Allergy Asthma Immunol* 74:415-418, 1995.

White IR, Lewis J, El Alami A: Possible adverse reactions to an enzyme-containing washing powder, *Contact Dermatitis* 13:175-179, 1985.

MACHINISTS

Job Description

Machinists set up and operate metal-cutting machines (Figure 15-9), including lathes, milling machines, sharpeners, and grinders that require metalworking fluids for lubrication and cooling.

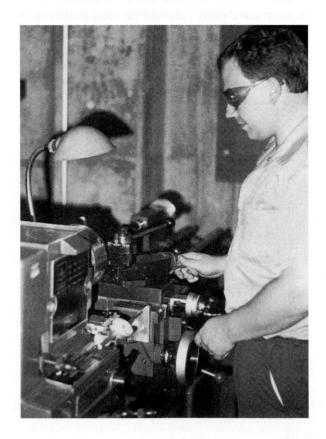

FIGURE 15-9
A machinist operating a lathe that requires metalworking fluids for lubrication and cooling. The metalworking fluid can cause irritant or allergic contact dermatitis.

Clinical Aspects

Virtually all manufactured products are constructed with tools or equipment made by machinists.

Preparation of the raw material and execution of the finishing touches require manual work at the workbench, including the use of hand tools, such as files and scrapers, which naturally involve friction and pressure on the worker's hands.

Metalworking fluids are a universal requirement to cool and lubricate the machine operation. These fluids are classified as insoluble, or neat, oils and water-based fluids (Table 15-2). Neat oils contain no water and are composed of mineral, fatty, or synthetic oils. In addition, they contain extreme-pressure additives, corrosion inhibitors, antifoam agents, dyes, and fragrances. Water-containing metalworking fluids include (1) soluble oils, which contain more than 50% mineral oil before emulsification; (2) semisynthetic fluids, which contain less than 50% mineral oil before emulsification; and (3) synthetic fluids, which contain no mineral oil but have polyalkylene glycol–type lubricants. Water-based metalworking fluids are more complex than the neat oils and contain preservatives, emulsifiers, and stabilizers, in addition to the other additives mentioned previously. Since the 1940s, there has been a change from neat oils to water-based fluids in many machining operations. With this, the incidence of oil folliculitis, oil acne, and skin cancer (from shale oil) has decreased, while the incidence of contact dermatitis has increased.

Metalworking fluids are the principal cause of contact dermatitis among machinists. It is usually considered to be chronic irritant dermatitis, mainly a result of the emulsifier (detergent, surfactant) component. A study of the irritancy of the metalworking fluids, however, found that they are generally only mildly irritant

Table 15-2	Contents of Metalworking Fluids
Insoluble (Neat) Oils	
Mineral oil	
Extreme-pressure additives	
Corrosive inhibitors	
Antifoaming agents	
Dyes	
Fragrances	
Soluble Oils, Semisynthetic and Synthetic Fluids	
Mineral oil (except synthetic fluids)	
Extreme-pressure additives	
Corrosive inhibitors	
Antifoaming agents	
Dyes	
Fragrances	
Water	
Emulsifiers	
Stabilizers	
Preservatives	

Kanerva L, Jolanki R, Estlander T et al: Incidence rates of occupational allergic contact dermatitis caused by metals, *Am J Contact Dermat* 11:155-160, 2000.

Mackey SA, Marks JG: Dermatitis in machinists: a retrospective study, *Am J Contact Dermat* 4:22-26, 1993.

Madden SD, Thiboutot DM, Marks JG: Occupationally induced allergic contact dermatitis to methylchloroisothiazolinone/methylisothiazolinone among machinists, *J Am Acad Dermatol* 30:272-274, 1994.

Mathias CGT: Contact dermatitis and metalworking fluids. In Byers JP, editor: *Metalworking fluids,* New York, 1994, Marcel Dekker.

Pryce DW, Irvine D, English JSC et al: Soluble oil dermatitis: a follow-up study, *Contact Dermatitis* 21:28-35, 1989.

Pryce DW, White J, English JSC et al: Soluble oil dermatitis: a review, *J Soc Occup Med* 39:93-98, 1989.

Robertson MH, Storrs FJ: Allergic contact dermatitis in two machinists, *Arch Dermatol* 118:997-1002, 1982.

Rossmoore HW: Antimicrobial agents for water-based metalworking fluids, *J Occup Med* 23:247-254, 1981.

Wigger-Alberti W, Krebs A, Elsner P: Experimental irritant contact dermatitis due to cumulative epicutaneous exposure to sodium lauryl sulphate and toluene: single and concurrent application, *Br J Dermatol* 143:551-556, 2000.

MECHANICS

Job Description

Mechanics repair cars (Figure 15-10), trucks, buses, and heavy equipment. They do routine maintenance such as lubrication, oil changes, tire rotation, engine tune-ups, and coolant system flushing. They also rebuild the engine and drive train and make other major repairs.

Clinical Aspects

Automotive mechanics are exposed to many irritants and allergens. The hands of an automobile mechanic are readily recognized by the residual grease and grime that collect under the fingernails and in the fissures and cracks of their hands. Mechanics are exposed to irritating fuels, cleansers, and solvents and often clean up with gasoline and abrasive soaps. Allergens are found in plastic materials that make up steering wheels, rubber chemicals in hoses and tires, additives to lubricants and fuels, and antifreeze.

Prevention

Because of the manual dexterity required, wearing protective gloves is usually impossible. The mechanic must be instructed not to use solvents, fuels, and abrasive soaps to clean his or her hands. Waterless hand soap is a better choice to remove grease. This should be followed by washing with a mild soap.

Irritants and Allergens

Irritants
    Solvents
    Cleaners
    Fuels

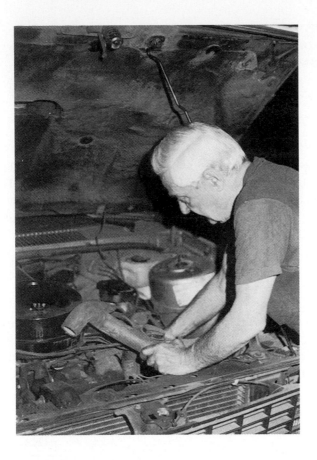

FIGURE 15-10
An automobile mechanic replacing a black rubber radiator hose, which contains allergens detected by the black rubber mix or *N*-isopropyl-*N*ꞌ-phenyl-*p*-phenylenediamine.

Fluids (brake, transmission, hydraulic, cooling)
Greases
Abrasive soaps and detergents
Allergens
    Standard tray
        Rubber chemicals (tires, hoses, gaskets, lubricants, antifreeze)
        p-Phenylenediamine (dyes in fuels)
        Potassium dichromate (cleaners, greases, gaskets, primers)
        Colophony (soldering flux)
        Epoxy (adhesives and sealants)
    Supplemental trays
        Antimicrobials, preservatives (Trolab/Hermal): Additives to fuels and
            other fluids, personal care products
    Additional allergens: Propylene glycol (Trolab/Hermal, Chemotechnique
        Diagnostics AB): Antifreeze

The most common allergens for mechanics are in the standard tray.

BIBLIOGRAPHY

Adams RM: *Occupational skin disease,* ed 2, Philadelphia, 1990, WB Saunders.

Meding B, Barregard L, Marcus K: Hand eczema in car mechanics, *Contact Dermatitis* 30:129-134, 1994.

MEDICAL WORKERS

Job Description

Medical workers are physicians, nurses, medical assistants, and technicians who work in hospitals, clinics, private offices, and nursing homes. They perform a wide range of jobs in providing health care. Therefore it is important to become familiar with the specific task that a health care provider does. It may be in the operating room as an orthopedic surgeon putting in artificial joints or in a nursing home as an aide providing skin care to bedridden patients.

Clinical Aspects

Health care personnel are particularly at risk for hand eczema; up to 40% of hospital employees are affected. A history of atopic dermatitis, previous disposition toward hand eczema, and wet work were predisposing risk factors. Irritant contact dermatitis from frequent hand washing is particularly a problem for nursing and operating room personnel (Figure 15-11).

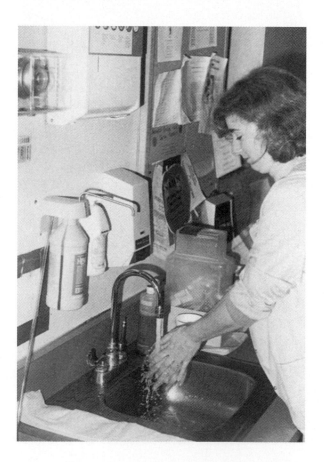

FIGURE 15-11
A neonatal intensive care nurse frequently washes her hands, which can cause irritant contact dermatitis.

Contact dermatitis and, more recently, contact urticaria to rubber gloves (Figure 15-12) have become prominent problems among medical personnel, since workers are using gloves more frequently to prevent transmission of the human immunodeficiency virus. Accelerators and antioxidants in rubber gloves are the most frequent contact sensitizers. A more insidious but probably more common problem is contact urticaria (see Chapter 16) from (powdered) natural rubber latex in gloves. The U.S. Occupational Safety and Health Administration estimates that 8% to 12% of health care workers are sensitized. Itching, erythema, and swelling develop within minutes of putting on gloves. The localized hand symptoms are sometimes associated with systemic symptoms such as rhinitis, conjunctivitis, wheezing, and faintness. After repeated episodes of contact urticaria, the physical examination of the hands reveals typical eczematous dermatitis that is incorrectly thought to result from contact dermatitis, not contact urticaria. The clinician diagnoses contact urticaria only with a high index of suspicion and direct questioning about the development of immediate symptoms. The history can be confirmed by radioallergosorbent test (RAST) testing or provocative skin tests with portions of the glove. Skin testing should be done cautiously, because anaphylaxis has occurred from immediate-type hypersensitivity reactions. Resuscitation equipment must be readily available.

> **Contact urticaria that is due to latex gloves should not be overlooked. Ask whether itching, erythema, and swelling develop within minutes of donning latex gloves.**

Glove powder may irritate skin areas covered by the glove and carries latex particles on its surface; therefore it enhances the probability of acquiring immediate-type latex allergy and latex protein contact dermatitis. Thus avoiding powered

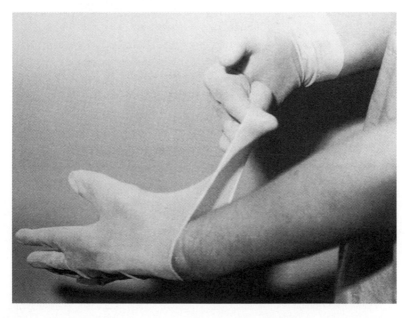

FIGURE 15-12
A medical worker donning rubber gloves, which can cause irritant or allergic contact dermatitis and contact urticaria.

gloves is a more certain way of preventing occupational skin disease in health professionals.

Glutaraldehyde (see Chapter 6) is a biocide commonly used in cold-sterilizing buffered solutions for disinfecting delicate medical instruments such as endoscopy (Figure 15-13) and uroscopy equipment, anesthetic gas machines, respirators, and renal dialysis apparatus; it is also used in x-ray solutions and embalming fluids. In a 5-year clinical patch test study at the University of Kansas, health care workers were found to be eight times more likely to be allergic to glutaraldehyde than their non–health care-working peers. Statistically relevant differences were also seen in their reactivity to thiomersal, benzalkonium chloride, and methyl methacrylate. Recent outbreaks of allergic contact dermatitis in health care workers have been attributed to glyoxal (ethynodiol), a dialdehyde disinfectant.

Orthopedic surgeons have allergic contact dermatitis that is due to the methyl methacrylate (see Chapter 7) in acrylic bone cement that is used to secure artificial joints. Surgical gloves provide little protection, since the methyl methacrylate monomer readily penetrates through these gloves. Besides causing allergic contact dermatitis, paresthesia of the fingertips has been produced.

Before disposable dispensers, medications were a prominent cause of allergic contact dermatitis in nursing personnel. Penicillin, sulfonamide, and mercurials were frequent allergens. Among psychiatric nurses, chlorpromazine and other related phenothiazine drugs caused allergic and photoallergic contact dermatitis.

Sensitization to inorganic mercury compounds may arise from liquid mercury released by broken thermometers. There are still topical disinfectants on the market that are based on organic mercury compounds. Thiomersal (merthiolate), an

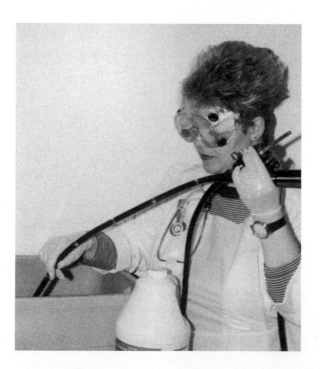

FIGURE 15-13
A nurse using a glutaraldehyde-buffered solution to cold-sterilize an endoscope. The glutaraldehyde can be an irritant or allergen.

organic mercury compound, is among the world's 10 most common contact allergens when routinely tested in a standard series.

Diammonium hydrogen phosphate, a flame retardant in surgical garb, was responsible for an outbreak of allergic contact dermatitis in surgical personnel.

Prevention

Infection control requires frequent hand washing. The use of barrier creams, mild soaps, and emollient creams may reduce irritant dermatitis. Contact dermatitis and contact urticaria from rubber gloves can be prevented with vinyl gloves or rubber gloves without the putative rubber allergen. Disposable medication cups, syringes, and cartridges significantly reduce contact with medications.

Manufacturers of acrylic bone cement recommend wearing two pairs of gloves and discarding them immediately after handling the cement. Because the acrylic monomers readily penetrate rubber surgical gloves, the effectiveness of double gloving in preventing dermatitis may be minimal. A "no-touch" technique should be used to mix and apply the cement.

Irritants and Allergens

Irritants
    Hand washing
    Gloves (occlusion, powder)
    Soaps, detergents
    Disinfectants
    Ethylene oxide
Allergens
    Standard tray
        Fragrances (skin care products)
        Rubber chemicals (gloves)
        Preservatives (hand creams, disinfectants)
        Potassium dichromate (chromic catgut)
    Supplemental trays
        Medicaments (Trolab/Hermal, Chemotechnique Diagnostics AB)
        Antimicrobials, preservatives, antioxidants (Trolab/Hermal): Glutaraldehyde, chlorhexidine diglucinate, benzalkonium chloride
        Vehicles, emulsifiers (Trolab/Hermal)
    Additional antigens
        Methyl methacrylate (Trolab/Hermal, Chemotechnique Diagnostics AB)
        Chlorpromazine hydrochloride (Trolab/Hermal, Chemotechnique Diagnostics AB)
        Povidone-iodine 10% solution
        Glyoxal 10% aqueous

> **The most common allergens in health care workers are:**
> 1. **Formaldehyde**
> 2. **Glutaraldehyde**
> 3. **Preservatives in skin care products, disinfectants**
> 4. **Mercaptobenzothiazole, tetramethylthiuram, and latex in gloves**

BIBLIOGRAPHY

Belsito DV: Contact dermatitis from diammonium hydrogen phosphate in surgical garb, *Contact Dermatitis* 23:267-268, 1990.

Berndt U, Wigger-Alberti W, Gabard B, Elsner P: Efficacy of a barrier cream and its vehicle as protective measures against occupational irritant contact dermatitis, *Contact Dermatitis* 42:77-80, 2000.

Camarasa JG: Health personnel. In Rycroft RJG, Menné T, Frosch PJ, editors: *Textbook of contact dermatitis,* Berlin, 1995, Springer-Verlag.

Cheng L, Lee D: Review of latex allergy, *J Am Board Fam Pract* 12:285-292, 1999.

Elsner P, Pevny I, Burg G: Occupational contact dermatitis due to glyoxal in health care workers, *Am J Contact Dermat* 1:250-253, 1990.

Fisher AA: Allergic dermatoses in the medical profession, *Immunol Allergy Clin North Am* 9:535-542, 1989.

Fisher AA: Allergic contact reactions in health personnel, *J Allergy Clin Immunol* 90:729-738, 1992.

Fowler JF: Allergic contact dermatitis from glutaraldehyde exposure, *J Occup Med* 31:852-853, 1989.

Gebhardt M: Health professions. In Gebhardt M, Elsner P, Marks JG, editors: *Handbook of contact dermatitis,* London, 2000, Dunitz.

Holness DL, Tarlo SM, Sussman G, Nethercott JR: Exposure characteristics and cutaneous problems in operating room staff, *Contact Dermatitis* 32:352-358, 1995.

Marks JG, Rainey MA: Cutaneous reactions to surgical preparations and dressings, *Contact Dermatitis* 10:1-5, 1984.

Nilsson E: Individual and environmental risk factors for hand eczema in hospital workers, *Acta Derm Venereol (Stockh)* 128:1-53, 1986.

Rudzki E, Rebandel P, Grzywa Z: Patch tests with occupational contactants in nurses, doctors, dentists, *Contact Dermatitis* 20:247-250, 1989.

Shaffer MP, Belsito DV: Allergic contact dermatitis from glutaraldehyde in health care workers, *Contact Dermatitis* 43:150-156, 2000.

Stingeni L, Lapomarda V, Lisi P: Occupational hand dermatitis in hospital environments, *Contact Dermatitis* 33:172-176, 1995.

Toraason M, Sussman G, Biagini R et al: Latex allergy in the workplace, *Toxicol Sci* 58:5-14, 2000.

OFFICE WORKERS

Job Description

Office personnel are employed predominantly in managerial and clerical positions. Their activities include preparing, transcribing, systematizing, and preserving written and oral communications. Their duties include stenography, typing, filing, programming, copying, and telephoning.

Clinical Aspects

The office is traditionally thought of as a clean, nonhazardous workplace. This to a large extent is true. Cutaneous problems among office workers, however, do occur. Suspected causes of these dermatoses include poor building ventilation, visual display terminals (VDTs), paper, and other miscellaneous office supplies and equipment.

The *sick-* or *tight-building syndrome* is a clustering of worker illness complaints found in modern energy-efficient buildings. These buildings limit the entry of fresh, outside air to reduce the cost of heating and cooling. Most commonly reported are symptoms of nose, eye, and throat irritation; dry skin; rashes; headache; and fatigue. This symptom complex can be quite distressing to the worker and result in epidemics of psychogenic illness. In most cases no specific air contaminants are found. It is important, however, that identifiable organic causes of the workers' complaints be ruled out. Otherwise, in some, *multiple chemical sensitivities* may evolve, characterized by multiorgan symptoms that are elicited by low-level exposure to chemicals of diverse structural classes in response to predictable stimuli and in which no standard test can explain symptoms.

Visual display terminals are a necessary part of the computer revolution that has occurred in the office (Figure 15-14). Musculoskeletal and visual complaints are the two most common problems reported by VDT workers and are usually controlled when attention is paid to ergonomics in workplace design and layout. Although there is no evidence that the radiation emitted from VDTs is harmful, considerable concern has arisen over the possibility of these units causing significant skin disease, particularly exacerbation of rosacea, seborrheic dermatitis, and acne. Lidén (1990) concluded that office workers, partly influenced by the mass media, wrongly blame VDTs for their skin problems.

Where would an office be without *paper*? Cases of allergic contact dermatitis on the basis of colophony allergy in which paper handling was a contributory cause have been reported. With the introduction of carbonless copy paper, complaints concerning handling paper increased. Allergic contact dermatitis is an uncommon reaction from carbonless copy paper. A second, much more common reaction is irritation of the skin and mucous membranes. Reported symptoms include itching and redness of the skin; burning of the eyes, nose, mouth, and chest; hoarseness; fatigue; headache; and nausea. Contact urticaria and upper

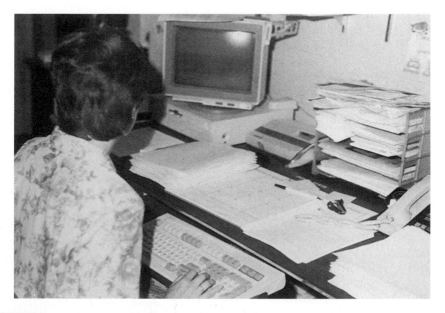

FIGURE 15-14
A secretary typing a manuscript at a Visual Display Terminal (VDT). Radiation from VDTs has been wrongly accused of exacerbating acne, rosacea, and seborrheic dermatitis.

airway obstruction have been observed to be due to carbonless copy paper. Other papers have also caused dermatoses in office workers: leukocytoclastic vasculitis from behenic acid in heat-activated photocopy paper, allergic contact dermatitis from a modified phenol formaldehyde maleic anhydride resin in type-writer correction paper, and allergic and photoallergic contact dermatitis from thiourea in photocopy paper.

> **The most frequent cause of office worker cutaneous complaints is *carbonless copy paper*. These are usually due to irritant contact dermatitis but may be due to contact urticaria or allergic contact dermatitis.**

Prevention

Good ventilation systems prevent "stale" air. Attention to ergonomics is important to the office workers who use a computer. Avoiding specific types of paper may prevent contact dermatitis and urticaria.

Irritants and Allergens

Irritants
    Wear and tear, friction
    Low humidity
    Carbonless copy paper
    Poor ventilation
    Solvents and cleaners
    Glues
    Toners
    Correcting fluids
Allergens
    Standard tray
        Nickel (scissors, paper clips)
        Formaldehyde (paper, glues)
        Rubber compounds (rubber bands, erasers)
        Colophony (paper)
    Additional allergens: Paper (as is)

BIBLIOGRAPHY

Bergqvist U, Wahlberg JE: Skin symptoms and disease during work with visual display terminals, *Contact Dermatitis* 30:197-204, 1994.

Eriksson N, Hoog J, Sandstrom M, Stenberg B: Facial skin symptoms in office workers: a five-year follow-up study, *J Occup Environ Med* 39:108-118, 1997.

Fiedler N, Maccia C, Kipen H: Evaluation of chemically sensitive patients, *J Occupational Med* 34:529-538, 1992.

Kanerva L, Estlander T, Jolanki R, Henriks-Eckerman ML: Occupational allergic contact dermatitis caused by diethylenetriamine in carbonless copy paper, *Contact Dermatitis* 29:147-151, 1993.

Karlberg A-T, Gäfvert E, Lidén C: Environmentally friendly paper may increase risk of hand eczema in rosin-sensitive persons, *J Am Contact Dermat* 33:427-432, 1995.

Lidén C: Contact allergy: a cause of facial dermatitis among visual display unit operators, *Am J Contact Dermat* 1:171-176, 1990.

Marks JG: Allergic contact dermatitis from carbonless copy paper, *JAMA* 245:2331-2332, 1981.

Marks JG: Dermatologic problems of office workers, *Dermatol Clin* 6:75-79, 1988.

Marks JG, Trautlein JJ, Zwillich CW et al: Contact urticaria and airway obstruction from carbonless copy paper, *JAMA* 252:1038-1040, 1984.

Thestrup-Pedersen K, Bach B, Petersen R: Allergic investigations in patients with the sick-building syndrome, *Contact Dermatitis* 23:53-55, 1990.

Wahlberg JE: Office environment, *Clin Dermatol* 15:587-592, 1997.

Whorton MD, Larson SR, Gordon NJ et al: Investigation and work-up of tight-building syndrome, *J Occup Med* 29:142-147, 1987.

PHOTOGRAPHERS

Job Description

Photographers and film laboratory workers develop film and print photographs through a succession of chemical baths containing developers, fixers, and rinses (Figure 15-15).

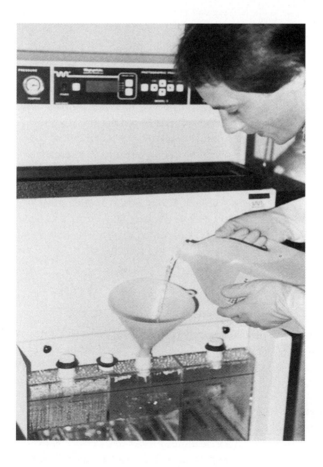

FIGURE 15-15
A photographer adding chemicals to a film-developing machine. Allergic contact dermatitis occurs from black-and-white (metol) and color (CD-2, CD-3) film developers.

Clinical Aspects

Despite a large amount of automation in film laboratories, workers still have contact with photographic chemicals. Lidén found that 21 (49%) of 43 of those working with photographic chemicals in a film laboratory had occupational dermatoses. Twelve (28%) had contact allergies to CD-2, CD-3, persulfate bleach accelerator–1 (PBA-1), or metol. Lichenoid eruptions were seen in two workers.

Contact dermatitis and lichenoid reactions to the color developers CD-2 and CD-3 are well known. Why exposure to these developers gives rise to dermatitis in some cases and a lichenoid reaction in others is unclear. CD-2, CD-3, and CD-4 are extremely potent sensitizers that cross-react with each other but not with *p*-phenylenediamine. Persulfate bleach accelerator–1 is an isothiouronium salt that is used for the development of color motion picture film. Metol (4-methylaminophenol sulfate) is the primary allergen in black-and-white film developers.

Contact vitiligo may be produced by developers containing hydroquinone. Only sporadic cases, however, have been reported in photography workers, probably because a low concentration of hydroquinone is used in film developers.

> **The most common photographic allergens are:**
> 1. **Metol (black-and-white film developer)**
> 2. **CD-2 and CD-3 color developers**

Prevention

Protective gloves should be used conscientiously to avoid skin contact with photographic chemicals. Worker education and automation also reduce potential risks.

Irritants and Allergens

Irritants
    Wet work
    Developers
    Fixers
    Bleaches
Allergens
    Standard tray
        Rubber chemicals (gloves)
        Ethylenediamine (developers)
        Formaldehyde (hardeners, developers)
        Potassium dichromate (cleaners, intensifiers)
    Supplemental trays: Photographic chemicals (Trolab/Hermal, Chemotechnique Diagnostics AB)

BIBLIOGRAPHY

Brancaccio RR, Cockerell CJ, Belsito D, Ostreicher R: Allergic contact dermatitis from color film developers: clinical and histologic features, *J Am Acad Dermatol* 28:827-830, 1993.

Brandao FM, Dinis A, Silva R: Contact dermatitis and vitiligo due to color developers. In Frosch PJ et al, editors: *Current topics in contact dermatitis,* Berlin, 1989, Springer-Verlag.

Lidén C: Occupational dermatoses at a film laboratory, *Contact Dermatitis* 10:77-87, 1984.

Lidén C, Bowman A, Sollenberg J: Color developing agents: high-performance liquid chromatography analysis of test preparations used in guinea pig maximization testing. In Frosch PJ et al, editors: *Current topics in contact dermatitis,* Berlin, 1989, Springer-Verlag.

Rustemeyer T, Frosch PJ: Allergic contact dermatitis from colour developers, *Contact Dermatitis* 32:59-60, 1995.

PRINTERS

Job Description

Most workers in the printing industry operate offset printing presses (Figure 15-16). Offset printing entails transferring an image with ink from the printing plate to an interposed rubber roller or blanket and then onto the printing stock. The printing plate image is made by a platemaker using a photographic process. The press operator sets up, adjusts, cleans, and repairs the printing press. He or she loads the machine with stock and ink and removes the printed material. Other printing systems include relief, gravure, and silk screen.

Clinical Aspects

The press worker has the greatest risk of irritant contact dermatitis resulting from the solvents that are used to clean the offset press. *Blanket washes* are composed

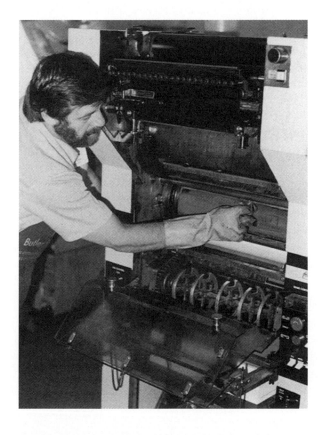

FIGURE 15-16
An offset printer cleaning the press with blanket wash, which contains solvents that can cause irritant contact dermatitis.

of aliphatic solvents such as methyl ethyl ketone, naphtha, or mineral spirits. *Wash-up solutions* are made of aromatic hydrocarbons such as toluene and acetone. A *fountain solution* composed of gum arabic, solvents, and acid in low concentration is used to wet the printing plate before it is inked. The printing *stock* may be paper, metal, or plastic, which is a rare cause of contact dermatitis.

Printing inks are composed of pigments dispersed in a vehicle plus various additives. The thicker inks such as those used in offset work contain linseed or other volatile petroleum, vegetable, or animal-based oils combined with natural colophony or synthetic (formaldehyde or phenolic derivative) resins. Recently developed nonvolatile inks are made of synthetic polymers such as epoxy acrylate, urethane acrylate, polyester acrylate, and multifunctional acrylic monomers (pentaerythritol triacrylate, hexanediol diacrylate, trimethylolpropane triacrylate). The polymerization of these acrylated resins is based on light-catalyzed cross-linkage of the polymers with monomers, and this results in drying of the ink. A light-absorbing chemical such as benzophenone is added to the ink to absorb the light from a high-intensity fluorescent ultraviolet lamp. The ultraviolet-cured acrylate ink monomers have caused allergic contact dermatitis. The same technology that is used to make ultraviolet-cured acrylate inks is also used to make printing plates. Exposure of printing factory workers to the photosensitive prepolymers in the printing plate or to solutions containing the uncured monomer produce a significant amount of sensitization. Fully cured plates do not represent a hazard.

Recent mortality studies found an increased occurrence of melanoma in the printing industry.

Prevention

Prevention of irritant contact dermatitis requires avoiding direct skin exposure to solvents that are used on the printing press. Wearing protective gloves and aprons while cleaning the machines is a must. For ultraviolet-cured acrylic resins, nitrile latex gloves provide adequate protection for an 8-hour work shift but are not reusable the following day. This is a rather expensive form of worker protection. The newer 4-H glove is an excellent barrier against epoxy and methacrylate monomers and may be the best glove for protection against these compounds.

Irritants and Allergens

Irritants
> Wet work
> Solvents (blanket wash, fountain solution)
> Inks
> Abrasive soaps and cleaners
> Desensitizing solutions
> Electrostatic solutions
> Greases and waxes
> Gum arabic
> UV light

Allergens
> Standard tray
>>   Preservatives (fountain solutions)
>>   Potassium dichromate (fountain solutions)

Rubber chemicals (gloves)
p-Phenylenediamine (ink)
Epoxy resin (ink)
Colophony (ink)
p-tert-Butylphenol formaldehyde resin (ink)
Supplemental trays
Antimicrobials, preservatives (Trolab/Hermal): Fountain solutions
(Meth)acrylate (Chemotechnique Diagnostics AB): Ultraviolet-cured inks and printing plates
Photographic chemicals (Trolab/Hermal, Chemotechnique Diagnostics AB): Photographic platemaking operation
Additional allergens: Printing ink (oil-based, as is; ultraviolet-cured, 1% in petrolatum)

The most frequent allergens in printers are:
1. **Potassium dichromate**
2. **Ink and printing plate resins**

BIBLIOGRAPHY

Emmett EA: Contact dermatitis from polyfunctional acrylic monomers, *Contact Dermatitis* 3:245-248, 1977.

Isaac MA, Thiboutot DM, Vasily DB, Marks JG: Contact dermatitis from printing inks, *Am J Contact Dermat* 3:142-144, 1992.

Mc Laughlin JK, Malker HS, Blot WJ et al: Malignant melanoma in the printing industry, *Am J Ind Med* 13:301-304, 1988.

Nethercott JR: Dermatitis in the printing industry, *Dermatol Clin* 6:61-66, 1988.

Nielsen H, Henriksen L, Olsen JH: Malignant melanoma among lithographers, *Scand J Work Environ Health* 22:108-111, 1996.

Rietschel RL: Contact allergens in ultraviolet-cured resin systems, *Occup Med* 1:301-306, 1986.

TEXTILE WORKERS

Job Description

Carding, spinning, weaving, dying, and finishing fabrics are to a large part mechanized in textile factories with little worker contact. Cutting and sewing fabrics to make clothing, on the other hand, are still done manually (Figure 15-17).

Clinical Aspects

Textile fibers are derived from animal (wool, silk), vegetable (flax, cotton), or synthetic (e.g., nylon, polyester, acrylic, spandex, saran) origin. The fibers are treated with a number of agents. The most important causes of contact dermatitis are the dyes and the resin finishes.

Of all the available textile fibers, only wool, silk, nylon, fiberglass, spandex, and rubber have been linked to cutaneous reactions. Irritant contact dermatitis most commonly results from wool and fiberglass. Although allergic contact dermatitis to nylon is most often due to a dye or finish, there have been reports of sensitivity to the nylon fiber itself. The allergen is probably a low-molecular-weight

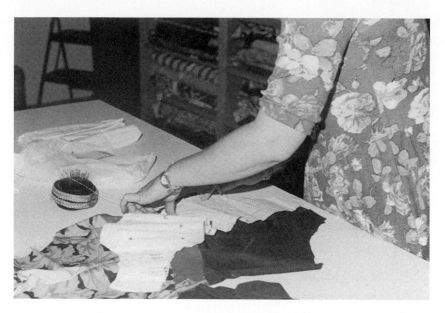

FIGURE 15-17
A textile worker pinning patterns on fabric before cutting. Allergic contact dermatitis may result from fabric dyes or resins.

polymer. Allergic contact dermatitis to spandex was traced to mercaptobenzothiazole added to the fiber-spinning bath. Mercaptobenzothiazole and thiuram allergies have been linked to rubber in bras, girdles, and other underwear. In several cases allergic contact dermatitis resulting from underwear occurred from an allergen produced when elastic rubber containing the accelerator zinc dibenzyldithiocarbamate was laundered with hypochlorite bleach. Contact urticaria has been reported from wool, silk, and nylon.

> **The most common textile allergens are:**
> 1. Dyes
> 2. Resins

The main dye sensitizers in textiles are azo dyes of the disperse type. These, however, are an uncommon cause of allergic contact dermatitis. The vast number of dyes, their many trade names, and their two types of classifications based on their *chemistry* (azo, anthraquinone, azine, indigoide, nitro, quinoline, triarylmethane, diphenylmethane, polyazo) or their *application method* (disperse, basic, acid, premetallic, reactive, direct, sulfur naphthols, vat) make comprehension of textile dyes complex. Also, new coloring agents are continuously introduced to the market; thus a close relationship with the textile industry is necessary to improve diagnostic tools. The azo and anthraquinone chemical dyes are sensitizers. Azo dyes, which may cross-react with *p*-phenylenediamine, account for 40% of all textile dyes. When classified by the method in which they are applied to textiles, these same azo and anthraquinone dyes are usually found in the disperse and reactive classes. Disperse Blue 106 (which cross-reacts with Disperse Blue 124) and *p*-phenylenediamine identify most individuals sensitive to dyes. The azo dyes—Disperse Yellow 3, Disperse Orange 3, Disperse Blue 124, and Disperse Red 1—are the most frequent sensitizers and have been combined in a screening disperse dye mix. Potassium dichromate used as a mordant to fasten dye to the fabric was responsible for an epidemic of allergic contact dermatitis among workers who manufacture blankets.

> ### *p*-Phenylenediamine and Disperse Blue 106 identify most cases of dye allergy.

Formaldehyde (see Chapter 5) and *N*-methylol compounds that are used to produce durable-press fabrics are an occasional cause of allergic contact dermatitis. Some individuals are sensitive to formaldehyde and some to the resin itself. Ureas, cyclic ureas, melamines, methylol carbamates, urons, and triazones are reacted with formaldehyde to form cross-links between adjacent cellulose molecules. This results in a durable-press, wrinkle-resistant finish. Investigations of marketplace fabrics in the United States and Europe during the 1960s and 1970s, when urea and melamine formaldehyde resins were the most frequently used, found up to 12,000 ppm free formaldehyde. The introduction of dimethylol dihydroxyethylene urea (DMDHEU) and its derivatives, today's most common fabric resin, resulted in much lower levels of free formaldehyde (i.e., in the range of 300 to 500 μg of formaldehyde per gram of fabric). The liberation of free formaldehyde from fabrics has been limited by law in Japan to a maximum of 75 ppm. In general, laundering wash-and-wear fabrics before wearing is recommended to reduce the formaldehyde. The use of chlorine bleach with laundering should be avoided, since this may increase formaldehyde release. Although formaldehyde patch testing identifies the majority of individuals who are allergic to textile resin finishes, the specific resin should also be tested.

> ### Ethylene urea/melamine formaldehyde resin mix (Fixapret ACO) is the best screening allergen for textile resin sensitivity.

Prevention

Mechanization of textile factories reduces the incidence of contact dermatitis significantly. Protective clothing should be worn when exposure to allergenic chemicals cannot be avoided.

Irritants and Allergens

Irritants
  Acids
  Alkalies
  Solvents
  Bleaches
  Fiberglass
  Detergents

Allergens
- Standard tray
  - Potassium dichromate (mordant)
  - Rubber chemicals (rubberized textiles)
  - Epoxy resin (adhesive)
  - *p*-Phenylenediamine (dyes)
  - Formaldehyde (resin finishes)
  - Nickel sulfate (tools)
- Supplemental trays
  - Textile colors and finish (Chemotechnique Diagnostics AB)
  - Textile dyes (Hermal/Trolab)
- Additional allergens: Fabric soaked in water and patch tested for 3 to 4 days (usually positive for a dye allergy but frequently negative for a resin allergy)

BIBLIOGRAPHY

Andersen KE, Hamann K: Cost benefit of patch testing with textile finish resins, *Contact Dermatitis* 8:64-67, 1982.

Belsito DV: Textile dermatitis, *Am J Contact Dermat* 4:249-252, 1993.

Cronin E: *Contact dermatitis,* Edinburgh, 1980, Churchill Livingstone.

Dooms-Goossens A: Textile dye dermatitis, *Contact Dermatitis* 27:321-323, 1992.

Estlander T, Kanerva L, Jolanki R: Occupational allergic dermatoses from textile, leather, and fur dyes, *Am J Contact Dermat* 1:13-20, 1990.

Fowler JF, Skinner SM, Belsito DV: Allergic contact dermatitis from formaldehyde resins in permanent press clothing: an underdiagnosed cause of generalized dermatitis, *J Am Acad Dermatol* 27:962-968, 1992.

Francalanci S, Angelini G, Balato N et al: Effectiveness of disperse dyes mix in detection of contact allergy to textile dyes: an Italian multicentre study, *Contact Dermatitis* 33:351, 1995.

Hatch KL, Maibach HI: Textile dye dermatitis: a review, *J Am Acad Dermatol* 12:1079-1092, 1985.

Hatch KL, Maibach HI: Textile fiber dermatitis, *Contact Dermatitis* 12:1-11, 1985.

Hatch KL, Maibach HI: Textile chemical finish dermatitis, *Contact Dermatitis* 14:1-3, 1986.

Hatch KL, Maibach HI: Textile dye dermatitis, *J Am Acad Dermatol* 32:631-639, 1995.

Hatch KL, Maibach HI: Textile dermatitis: an update. I. Resins, additives and fibers, *Contact Dermatitis* 32:319-326, 1995.

Hatch KL, Maibach HI: Textile dye allergic contact dermatitis prevalence, *Contact Dermatitis* 42:187-195, 2000.

Hausen BM: Contact allergy to Disperse Blue 106 and Blue 124 in black "velvet" clothes, *Contact Dermatitis* 28:169-173, 1993.

Hausen BM, Sawall EM: Sensitization experiments with textile dyes in guinea pigs, *Contact Dermatitis* 20:27-31, 1989.

Jordan WP, Bourlas MC: Allergic contact dermatitis to underwear elastic, *Arch Dermatol* 111:593-595, 1975.

Lisboa C, Barros A, Azenha A: Contact dermatitis from textile dyes, *Contact Dermatitis* 31:9-10, 1994.

Manzini BM, Motolese A, Conti A et al: Sensitization to reactive textile dyes in patients with contact dermatitis, *Contact Dermatitis* 34:172-175, 1996.

Sadhra S, Duhra P, Foulds IS: Occupational dermatitis from synacril red 3B liquid (C1 basic red 22), *Contact Dermatitis* 21:316-320, 1989.

Seidenari S, Manzini BM, Danese P: Contact sensitization to textile dyes: description of 100 subjects, *Contact Dermatitis* 24:253-258, 1991.

Seidenari S, Manzini BM, Schiavi ME, Motolese A: Prevalence of contact allergy to non-disperse azo dyes for natural fibers: a study in 1814 consecutive patients, *Contact Dermatitis* 33:118-122, 1995.

Sertoli A, Francalanci S, Giorgini S: Sensitization to textile disperse dyes: validity of reduced-concentration patch tests and a new mix, *Contact Dermatitis* 31:47-48, 1994.

Sherertz EF: Contact dermatitis in textile industry workers, *Am J Contact Dermat* 2:69, 1991.

Sherertz EF: Clothing dermatitis: practical aspects for the clinician, *Am J Contact Dermat* 3:55-64, 1992.

Soni BP, Sherertz EF: Contact dermatitis in the textile industry: a review of 72 patients, *Am J Contact Dermat* 7:226-230, 1996.

Storrs FJ: Dermatitis from clothing and shoes. In Fisher AA, editor: *Contact dermatitis,* ed 3, Philadelphia, 1986, Lea & Febiger.

PART IV

Additional Topics

CHAPTER 16

Contact Urticaria

DEFINITION

Contact urticaria is a transient, wheal-and-flare response at the site of cutaneous contact to a topically applied material. Lesions occur within minutes to an hour, resolve within a few hours, and leave normal skin. A greater understanding of contact urticaria led to a broader concept of this phenomenon that included a spectrum of reactions from a weak suburticarial form manifested by erythema to the contact urticarial syndrome that has urticaria and systemic anaphylactic symptoms. A great number of agents produce contact urticaria, including foods, fragrances, flavorings, medicaments, metals, animal and plant products, preservatives and disinfectants, industrial chemicals, and physical agents. The prevalence of contact urticaria among the general population is unknown, but it may be a relatively common and underrecognized condition. A detailed patient history with attention to the rapid onset of symptoms suggests a contact urticarial reaction.

PATHOGENESIS

Contact urticaria may be produced by immunologic or nonimmunologic mechanisms. The pathogenesis of immunologically mediated contact urticaria is better understood than nonimmunologic contact urticaria.

> **Immunologic (immunoglobulin E–mediated) and nonimmunologic mechanisms can produce contact urticaria.**

Immunologic contact urticaria is caused by an antigen antibody, type 1, immunoglobulin E (IgE)–mediated hypersensitivity reaction. The antigen is the chemical contactant that binds to specific IgE antibodies on the surface of dermal mast cells. This triggers degranulation and liberation of vasoactive substances, primarily histamine, that cause dermal edema surrounded by an erythematous flare. Elevated serum levels of specific IgE antibodies have been demonstrated in response to contact urticariogens such as natural latex. Other immunologic mechanisms that have been implicated in the wheal-and-flare response include IgM- and IgG-mediated activation of the complement cascade through the classic pathway. These latter mechanisms have not been confirmed in the contact urticaria response. Characteristically, individuals who have immunologic contact urticaria constitute a low proportion of the exposed subjects. They have had previous exposure to the contactant without symptoms (sensitization phase) before the development of contact urticaria (elicitation phase). Immunologic contact urticaria may become generalized and produce systemic anaphylactic reactions.

Nonimmunologic contact urticarial reactions are less well understood with regard to their pathogenesis. It appears that a variety of mediators may initiate the urticarial response, depending on the contactant. This requires no prior sensitization and is not antibody mediated. It is the most common type of contact urticaria and occurs in the majority of individuals exposed to the contactant. The reaction remains localized, in contrast to immunologically mediated urticaria. Nonimmunologic contact urticaria may result from a direct effect on dermal blood vessels or by the release of inflammatory mediators such as histamine, prostaglandins, leukotrienes, and substance P. Indomethacin and acetylsalicylic acid, known prostaglandin inhibitors, abolish the urticarial reaction caused by topically applied benzoic acid, cinnamic acid, cinnamic aldehyde, methyl nicotinate, and diethyl fumarate. On the other hand, the reaction is not inhibited by the antihistamines hydroxyzine or terfenadine. Topical capsaicin pretreatment inhibits erythema in the histamine prick test. But topical capsaicin did not have any distinct effect on the erythema caused by the nonimmunologic, immediate erythematous reactions to benzoic acid and methyl nicotinate. A topical anesthetic cream composed of lidocaine and prilocaine, however, inhibited the erythema and edema caused by benzoic acid, methyl nicotinate, and histamine. It is not known whether the inhibitory effect was due to the anesthetic cream's effect on cutaneous sensory nerves or some other regulatory mechanisms. Interestingly, ultraviolet light A and B inhibit nonimmunologic, immediate contact reactions to benzoic acid. The effect lasts for more than 2 weeks and is poorly understood.

CLINICAL ASPECTS

The range of contact urticaria reactions comprises a spectrum from localized cutaneous urticaria to involvement of extracutaneous organs. Maibach and Johnson (1975) called this spectrum the *contact urticaria syndrome* and divided it into the following stages: (1) localized urticaria restricted to the area of contact; (2) generalized urticaria including angioedema; (3) urticaria associated with bronchial asthma, rhinitis, and conjunctivitis and orolaryngeal and gastrointestinal tract symptoms; and (4) urticaria associated with anaphylactoid reactions. In their review of the literature, von Krogh and Maibach (1981) found that 15% of patients with contact urticaria also had a history suggesting extracutaneous symptoms involving the respiratory and gastrointestinal systems. Anaphylactoid reactions were uncommon. One third of the cases reported had associated generalized urticaria. Of interest, a number of patients had both immediate and delayed reactions: immediate contact urticaria followed 24 to 48 hours later by contact dermatitis. Nonimmunologically mediated contact urticaria rarely produces extracutaneous symptoms.

> **Contact Urticaria Syndrome Stages**
> 1. **Localized urticaria**
> 2. **Generalized urticaria**
> 3. **Urticaria plus asthma, eye, nose, mouth, and gastrointestinal tract symptoms**
> 4. **Urticaria plus anaphylactoid reactions**

There are some chemicals that are capable of producing either immunologic or nonimmunologic urticaria. There are also chemicals that cause contact urticaria, which has features of both immunologic and nonimmunologic mechanisms. For example, ammonium persulfate (used to boost permanent hair bleaches) sometimes causes contact urticaria as well as generalized reactions including asthma and syncope. Testing produced conflicting results as to whether this represents an immunologic or nonimmunologic reaction. Solar urticaria and aquagenic urticaria, when investigated, also produced results supporting both immunologic and nonimmunologic mechanisms.

The number of substances that have been reported to produce contact urticaria are protean. These may be well-defined chemicals such as formaldehyde or chemically poorly defined substances such as dog saliva. Several authors, such as Lahti and Maibach (1989) and Warner and others (1997) listed over 200 substances reported to cause contact urticaria. Some agents commonly cause contact urticaria. For example, benzoic acid, cinnamic acid, and sorbic acid caused contact urticaria in 88%, 85%, and 58% of subjects tested, respectively. These reactions represent nonimmunologic contact urticaria and are very frequently manifested by only localized erythema. Benzoic acid, sorbic acid, and sodium benzoate, used as preservatives for cosmetics and as flavoring agents in foods and drugs, can produce contact urticaria reactions at concentrations as low as 0.1% to 0.2%. Cinnamic aldehyde, a fragrance material, can elicit erythema and stinging at a concentration of 0.01%. This explains why some mouthwashes and chewing gums that contain cinnamic aldehyde produce a tingling sensation of the mouth. Higher concentrations can cause lip swelling and urticaria in normal skin. Arthropods, nettles, and marine life have long been known to trigger nonimmunologic contact urticaria. In these cases urticaria results from bites, fine hairs, spines, or stings that injure the skin and allow entry of urticariogenic agents.

> **Medicaments, foods, animal and plant products, cosmetic ingredients, metals, and industrial chemicals produce contact urticaria.**

Immunologically mediated contact urticaria has been proved to be caused by animal products including hair, urine, and saliva and by latex gloves, biocides, and foods. Fruits and vegetables such as apple, peach, potato, and carrot have caused itching, tingling, and edema of the hands, lips, tongue, and pharynx after handling and eating these foods. *Protein contact dermatitis* is a subset of contact urticaria that is used to describe individuals, particularly food workers, with hand eczema in whom symptoms of itching, erythema, urticarial swelling, and small vesicles developed within minutes of contact with food protein such as fish or shellfish. After repeated episodes of contact urticaria, some individuals exhibit a chronic dermatitis appearance.

Contact urticaria is common in occupational settings. Other than for latex, there is little statistical data on occupational contact urticaria. According to data reported from Finland, farmers have the most cases, and bakers have the highest rate. The authors found cow dander, natural rubber latex, flour, grains, and feed to be the most common causes (Kanerva, 1996).

TESTS

The diagnosis of contact urticaria is suspected by a history that reveals symptoms within minutes to an hour of skin contact and is confirmed with testing. Contact urticarial testing must be performed with resuscitation equipment readily available to manage potential anaphylactic reactions. The patient's history should suggest whether extracutaneous reactions are a significant hazard.

> **Testing for contact urticaria should be monitored carefully to treat potentially life-threatening anaphylactic reactions.**

The initial and simplest in vivo diagnostic test for contact urticaria is the open test. In this procedure, a small amount of the suspected material is applied (full strength or dissolved in the appropriate vehicle) to normal skin of the upper portion of the back or forearm. For convenience, the forearm is preferred. The test site is observed periodically for 60 minutes. If open testing on normal skin is negative, the test should be performed on slightly dermatitic or previously affected skin. Open testing is the safest method because of the low risk of anaphylaxis. There is no standard scoring system to grade contact urticarial reactions, which range from macular erythema to the wheal-and-flare response.

Closed or occlusive testing using a patch or chamber can be done when open testing results are negative. The closed test is said to be somewhat more sensitive because it causes greater penetration of the test material. The patch is removed after 15 to 20 minutes, and the test site (normal or dermatitic skin) observed for an additional 60 minutes. Routine patch testing, of course, misses a contact urticarial response, since the patches are removed at 48 hours, long after the urticaria has resolved.

Scratch, prick, or intradermal tests may be employed if the open or closed test results are negative. These tests are usually done for immunologically mediated contact urticarial reactions. They are particularly useful for allergens of high molecular weight such as food proteins. Patients must be monitored carefully during these test procedures, and the necessary equipment and personnel must be available to treat potentially life-threatening reactions, particularly in patients who, in addition to localized contact urticaria, have accompanying generalized urticaria with associated extracutaneous symptoms such as wheezing or abdominal cramping. Guidelines for standardizing diagnostic tests of IgE-dependent reactions have been outlined by Bernstein (1988). Kanerva and others (1991) have abandoned intradermal testing because of the risk of anaphylaxis. They provide detailed methods of prick, scratch, and scratch-chamber tests as performed by specially trained nurses. The prick technique of skin testing is done with a sterile disposable needle. A drop of the test material is placed on the skin, and the needle is passed through the drop at a 45-degree angle. The skin is penetrated and gently lifted. This creates a small break in the epidermis and, when done properly, no bleeding occurs. For scratch testing, a 5- to 10-mm long, superficial scratch without bleeding is made with a sterile disposable needle; then the putative allergen is applied to the scratch. Interpretation of prick and scratch test reactions requires evaluation of the wheal only. Histamine hydrochloride (10 mg/ml) and the test solution without antigen are used as positive and negative controls, respectively. A sufficient number of controls is required, especially with scratch and intradermal testing, because many materials produce positive reactions in a nonimmunologic manner.

> **Test procedures for Contact Urticaria**
> 1. **Open test: Normal or affected skin**
> 2. **Closed test: Normal or affected skin**
> 3. **Prick, scratch, or intradermal test**
> 4. **Radioallergosorbent test**

In vitro testing with the radioallergosorbent test (RAST) avoids the possibility of anaphylaxis. The RAST procedure involves coupling the allergen to cellulose particles or paper disks. The allergen-immunosorbent is then reacted with the patient's serum containing specific IgE antibodies. The amount of specific IgE reacting with the antigen is measured with radioactively labeled anti-IgE antibody. The RAST procedure is unavailable for many contact allergens.

A procedure that was previously used to confirm immunologically mediated contact urticaria is the passive transfer or Prausnitz-Küstner test. This entails injection of the patient's serum into the skin of a human volunteer. Twenty-four hours later, the contactant is topically applied to the injection site. A wheal-and-flare response indicates the presence of specific IgE antibodies in the test serum and an immunologic mechanism. Because of concerns about the potential of transferring infectious diseases such as hepatitis and the acquired immunodeficiency syndrome, passive transfer is not used anymore.

A skin biopsy, although in most cases unnecessary, confirms an urticarial lesion. It is not specific for the diagnosis of contact urticaria. The histopathologic appearance can range from mild dermal edema to a superficial, and deep perivascular mixed-cell infiltrate composed of eosinophils, neutrophils, mast cells, and lymphocytes. Older lesions often show dermal edema with eosinophils situated between collagen bundles.

MANAGEMENT

Prevention is the obvious mainstay in managing contact urticaria. Identification and avoidance of the offending substance is the best solution. Individuals with immunologic contact urticaria, in particular, should avoid the contact allergen, since repeated exposures may result in progressively worsening symptoms and possibly lead to anaphylaxis. When prevention fails, antihistamines have been traditionally used to reduce the urticarial symptoms. Hydroxyzine hydrochloride is the most effective in blocking the wheal-and-flare response. In cases of severe generalized urticaria, systemic glucocorticoids are often employed. For anaphylactic reactions, epinephrine, oxygen, and supportive emergency measures are required.

BIBLIOGRAPHY

Adinoff AD, Rosloniec DM, McCall LL et al: A comparison of six epicutaneous devices in the performance of immediate hypersensitivity skin testing, *J Allergy Clin Immunol* 84:168-174, 1989.

Amin S, Maibach HI: Contact urticaria syndrome: 1996, *Cosmetics Toiletries* 110:29-33, 1995.

Amin S, Tanglertsampan C, Maibach HI: Contact urticaria syndrome: 1997, *Am J Contact Dermat* 8:15-19, 1997.

Bernstein IL, editor: Relevant in vivo and in vitro diagnostic tests of IgE-dependent reactions (immediate hypersensitivity), *J Allergy Clin Immunol* 82:488-507, 1988.

Emmons WW, Marks JG: Immediate and delayed reactions to cosmetic ingredients, *Contact Dermatitis* 13:258-265, 1985.

Fisher AA, Dooms-Goossens A: Persulfate hair bleach reactions: cutaneous and respiratory manifestations, *Arch Dermatol* 112:1047, 1976.

Gollhausen R, Kligman AM: Human assay for identifying substances which include nonallergic contact urticaria: the NICU test, *Contact Dermatitis* 13:98-106, 1985.

Hannuksela M: Mechanisms in contact urticaria, *Clin Dermatol* 15:619-622, 1997.

Kanerva L, Estlander T, Jolanki R: Skin testing for immediate hypersensitivity in occupational allergology. In Menné T, Maibach H, editors: *Exogenous dermatoses: environmental dermatitis,* Boca Raton, Fla, 1991, CRC.

Kanerva L, Toikkanen J, Jolanki R, Estlander T: Statistical data on occupational contact urticaria, *Contact Dermatitis* 35:229-233, 1996.

Katchen B, Maibach HI: Immediate-type contact reaction: immunologic contact urticaria. In Menné T, Maibach H, editors: *Exogenous dermatoses: environmental dermatitis,* Boca Raton, Fla, 1991, CRC.

Kligman AM: The spectrum of contact urticaria: wheals, erythema, and pruritus, *Dermatol Clin* 8:57-60, 1990.

Lahti A: Nonimmunologic contact urticaria, *Acta Derm Venereol (Stockh)* 60(suppl 91):1-49, 1980.

Lahti A: Immediate contact reactions. In Rycroft RJG, Menné T, Frosch PJ, editors: *Textbook of contact dermatitis,* ed 2, Berlin, 1995, Springer-Verlag.

Lahti A, Maibach HI: Immediate contact reactions, *Immunol Allergy Clin North Am* 9:463-478, 1989.

Lahti A, Vaananen A, Kokkonen E et al: Acetylsalicylic acid inhibits nonimmunologic contact urticaria, *Contact Dermatitis* 16:133-135, 1987.

Maibach HI, Johnson HL: Contact urticaria syndrome: contact urticaria to diethyltoluamide (immediate-type hypersensitivity), *Arch Dermatol* 111:726-730, 1975.

Marks JG: Contact urticaria, *Cosmetics Toiletries* 101:59-62, 1986.

McDaniel WR, Marks JG: Contact urticaria due to sensitivity to spray starch, *Arch Dermatol* 115:628, 1979.

Rietschel RL, Fowler JF: *Fisher's contact dermatitis,* ed 4, Baltimore, 1995, Williams & Wilkins, pp 778-807.

Ryan MD, Davis BM, Marks JG: Contact urticaria and allergic contact dermatitis to benzocaine gel, *J Am Acad Dermatol* 2:221-223, 1980.

Skinner S, Fowler JF: Contact anaphylaxis: a review, *Am J Contact Dermat* 6:133-142, 1995.

von Krogh GV, Maibach HI: The contact urticaria syndrome: an updated review, *J Am Acad Dermatol* 5:328-342, 1981.

Wakelin SH: Contact urticaria, *Clin Exp Dermatol* 26:132-136, 2001.

Warner MR, Taylor JS, Leow YH: Agents causing contact urticaria, *Clin Dermatol* 15:623-635, 1997.

CONTACT URTICARIA

Rubber

Since Nutter (1979) reported a case of contact urticaria from rubber gloves, a number of individuals with contact urticaria and anaphylaxis to natural rubber (latex) have been described. Health care workers, rubber industry workers, and children with spina bifida or urogenital abnormalities are most at risk for latex allergy. At present, the incidence of NRL allergy is still unknown, but several prevalence studies have been published. In European health-care workers screened with prick test prevalences of 2.8 to 10, 7% were reported (Turjanmaa, 1987; Lagier and others, 1992). A recent serological study based on RAST found a 5.5% prevalence of NRL allergy among 381 investigated hospital workers (Kaczmarek and others, 1996). For children with spina bifida, who have shown the highest prevalence of NRL allergy, a frequency of up to 50% has been reported in prick screenings and serological IgE measurements (Kelly and others, 1993).

Among the general population the occurrence of NRL allergy has not been systematically investigated. However, it seems to range under the 2% level. In a study of 804 unselected adult Finns, only one person (0.12%) showed a NRL allergy when screened by prick test (Turjanmaa and others, 1995).

In addition to latex gloves, balloons, condoms, dental dams, and other rubber objects have been the etiologic agents. Itching and burning with or without localized contact urticaria when wearing rubber gloves are the most frequent symptoms. Less frequently, extracutaneous symptoms such as rhinitis, conjunctivitis, facial edema, and asthma are reported. Of greatest concern is severe anaphylactic reactions, which in some cases have been fatal. Exposure to latex antigen can occur by cutaneous, respiratory, mucosal, and parenteral routes; the latter two routes have the greatest risk of anaphylaxis.

Latex is the milky sap obtained from the rubber tree *Hevae brasiliensis.* It is filtered and then preserved with either ammonia or sodium sulfite. The liquid latex is useful for the manufacture of gloves, condoms, balloons, rubber adhesives, and other products. Natural latex contains proteins, lipids, amino acids, nucleotides, cofactors, and the abundant terpene polymer, *cis*-1,4-polyisoprene. It is *cis*-1,4-polyisoprene that is purified and cross-linked (vulcanization) by slow heating with sulfur to make *rubber.* The contact dermatitis allergens mercaptobenzothiazoles, thiurams, and dithiocarbamates are added as catalysts (accelerators) to speed up the vulcanization curing process. Phenylenediamine derivatives are added to increase durability as antioxidants. The latex allergens that cause immediate hypersensitivity appear to be water-soluble proteins with allergenic fractions having molecular weights ranging from 2 to 100 kilodaltons. Prohevein and hevein have been recently characterized to be major allergens for health-care workers, whereas Rubber Elongation Factor (REF) and a 27-kDa NRL protein are important allergens for children with a history of multiple surgical procedures (Alenius and others, 1994; Alenius and others, 1995; Alenius and others, 1996). The formation of neonantigens during the manufacturing process has also been suggested. The range of antigen content varies greatly in latex products. For example, there is at least a 3000-fold difference in different brands of gloves. Therefore the Food and Drug Administration (FDA) in the United States and the European Committee for Standardisation (CEN) have acknowledged the measurement of total protein as a simple option for monitoring NRL products. Thus consumers can be informed of highly allergenic glove brands in the market (Palosuo and others, 1997; Palosuo and others, 1998).

A water-soluble protein is the allergen in latex-induced contact urticaria.

Taylor and others (1990) reported 10 cases of contact urticaria from latex gloves and one from a latex condom. Seven had concomitant or preceding hand eczema, and two had allergic contact dermatitis resulting from latex gloves. Several had a history of contact urticaria from other latex items such as balloons and a dental dam. Use and prick and/or scratch test results were positive in all cases tested. Radioallergosorbent test findings were positive in five of eight cases. Two patients had anaphylactic reactions following mucosal contact with latex, one from surgical gloves, and the other from a condom.

Pecquet and others (1990) reported 17 women who had contact urticaria to natural latex. Twelve had an anaphylactic reaction during surgery, and five had contact urticaria. Prick tests done through washed surgical gloves were positive in 15 of 17 patients, and through natural latex they were positive in 16 of 16 patients. Radioallergosorbent test findings for specific latex IgE antibodies were positive in 12 of 17 cases.

Tarlo and others (1990) reported occupational asthma caused by latex in a surgical glove manufacturing plant. They found that 3 (3.7%) of 81 of the workers had latex-related asthma while working with the finished gloves. None of these three had known skin disease, unlike previously reported subjects with anaphylactic reactions to latex. The respiratory manifestations of their allergy suggested that exposure to the latex antigen was by inhalation, possibly in association with the glove powder.

Turjanmaa and others (1988a) compared several methods to make the diagnosis of latex surgical glove contact urticaria. They found that prick testing with a stock solution made from latex gloves yielded positive reactions in all 15 subjects. Prick testing with sap from the rubber tree *H. brasiliensis* was positive in 12 of 15. Scratch-chamber test responses to the crushed rubber tree leaf were positive in 13 of 15. A latex glove use test was positive in 12 of 13, and the RAST procedure positive in 8 of 15. The authors concluded that the use test with glove and/or prick tests with a latex surgical glove solution were adequate for diagnosing latex glove contact urticaria. Others have confirmed and expanded those findings. Kelly and others (1994) present an algorithm of diagnostic testing steps beginning with in vitro serum test and proceeding to in vivo use and skin tests.

> **The diagnosis of rubber contact urticaria is suspected from a history of immediate symptoms after exposure to rubber and confirmed with positive use or prick test results. Radioallergosorbent test findings are less frequently positive but this should be the initial test, to avoid anaphylaxis.**

The coexistence of an immediate and delayed rubber glove allergy is not infrequent. Turjanmaa and others (1988b) studied 53 glove-allergic patients, 35 with an immediate allergy to latex and 18 with delayed allergy to rubber chemicals. Of the immediate allergy patients, 5 (14%) of 35 had positive patch test responses to thiurams. Of the delayed allergy patients, 1 (6%) of 18 had a positive prick test to latex. Atopy and hand dermatitis appeared to be predisposing factors for the development of immediate allergy to latex.

> **Repeated contact urticaria from latex gloves can mimic the appearance of a chronic hand dermatitis.**

Belsito (1990) in his analysis of seven cases of contact urticaria caused by rubber makes the point that allergens other than natural latex can be the putative agent. Cornstarch powder, mercaptobenzothiazole, black rubber mix, and carbamates in rubber gloves and condoms were the contact urticaria allergens.

Patients with latex sensitivity may also have allergic reactions to banana, avocado, and other foods, which becomes evident as urticaria, oral itching, rhinitis, asthma, and anaphylaxis. Cross-reacting IgE antibodies in the sera of these patients have been demonstrated to common allergens in latex, banana, and avocado.

> **Banana, avocado, and other foods can cause allergic reactions in latex-sensitive individuals.**

Prevention of allergic reactions by avoiding latex may be difficult, considering the ubiquity of latex in medical, industrial, and household products and routes of exposure ranging from direct contact to aerosol spread. For example, cornstarch glove powder absorbs latex protein and can be easily aerosolized in surgical suites and laboratories. Premedication cannot be used as an alternative to careful antigen avoidance. Autoinjectable epinephrine should be carried by individuals with more severe reactions. Wearing a Medic-Alert identification bracelet and carrying nonlatex gloves are also recommended (Table 16-1). There are several possible routes of exposure to natural rubber during surgery. Anesthesiologists and surgeons should use nonlatex gloves, tubings, bottles, and other equipment such as breathing bags to avoid anaphylactic reactions. Surgical gloves that do not contain

Table 16-1	Nonlatex Gloves	
Brand Name	**Polymer**	**U.S. Source**
Surgical		
Tactyl 1 and 2	Copolymer	Allerderm
Neolon	Neoprene	Becton Dickinson
Dermaprene	Neoprene	Ansel
Elastyren	Styrene butadiene	Hermal
Examination		
Tactyl 1 and 2	Copolymer	Allerderm
SensiCare	Vinyl	Becton Dickinson
TruTouch	Vinyl	Becton Dickinson
Vinylite	Vinyl	SmartPractice
Flexam	Vinyl	Baxter
Baxter	Vinyl	Baxter
Meditouch	Vinyl	AMG Medical
Dispos-a-glove	Copolymer	Johnson & Johnson

natural latex include Elastyren, Neolon, Tactyl 1 and 2, and Dermaprene. Latex-free surgical suites have been developed in some medical centers.

BIBLIOGRAPHY

Alenius H, Kalkkinen N, Lukka M et al: Purification and partial amino acid sequencing of a 27 kD natural rubber allergen recognized by latex allergic children with spina bifida, *Int Arch Allergy Immunol* 106:258-262, 1994.

Alenius H, Kalkkinen N, Lukka M et al: Prohevein from the rubber tree *(Hevea brasiliensis)* is a major latex allergen, *Clin Exp Allergy* 25:659-665, 1995.

Alenius H, Kalkkinen N, Turjanmaa K et al: Significance of the rubber elongation factor as ala-tex allergen, *Int Arch Allergy Immunol* 109:362-368, 1996.

Belsito DW: Contact urticaria caused by rubber: analysis of seven cases, *Dermatol Clin* 8:61-66, 1990.

Blaiss MS: Latex allergy in children: a review, *Pediatr Asthma Allergy Immunol* 6:71-75, 1992.

Hamann CP: Natural rubber latex protein sensitivity in review, *Am J Contact Dermat* 4:4-21, 1993.

Kelly KJ, Kurup V, Zacharisen M et al: Skin and serologic testing in the diagnosis of latex allergy, *J Allergy Clin Immunol* 91:1140-1145, 1993.

Kelly KJ, Kurup VP, Reijula KE, Fink JN: The diagnosis of natural rubber latex allergy, *J Allergy Clin Immunol* 93:813-816, 1994.

Lavaud F, Prevost A, Cossart C et al: Allergy to latex, avocado, pear, and banana: evidence for a 30-kD antigen in immunoblotting, *J Allergy Clin Immunol* 95:557-540, 1995.

Lagier F, Vervloet D, Lhermet I et al: Prevalence of latex allergy in operating room nurses, *J Allergy Clin Immunol* 90:319-22,1992.

Mäkinen-Kijunen S: Banana allergy in patients with immediate-type hypersensitivity to natural rubber latex: characterization of cross-reacting antibodies and allergens, *J Allergy Clin Immunol* 93:990-996, 1994.

Nutter AF: Contact urticaria to rubber, *Br J Dermatol* 101:597-598, 1979.

Palosuo T, Turjanmaa K, Reinikka-Railo H: *Allergen content of latex gloves: a market surveillance study of medical gloves used in Finland in* 1997, Helsinki, 1997, National Agency for Medicines.

Palosuo T, Mäkinen-Kiljunen S, Alenius H et al: Measurement of natural rubber latex allergen levels in medical gloves by allergen-specific IgE-ELISA inhibition, RAST inhibition, and skin prick test, *Allergy* 53:59-67, 1998.

Pecquet C, Leynadier F, Dry J: Contact urticaria and anaphylaxis to natural latex, *J Am Acad Dermatol* 22:631-633, 1990.

Slater JE: Rubber anaphylaxis, *N Engl J Med* 320:1126-1130, 1989.

Slater JE: Latex allergy, *J Allergy Clin Immunol* 94:139-149, 1994.

Spaner D, Dolovich J, Tarlo S et al: Hypersensitivity to natural latex, *J Allergy Clin Immunol* 83:1135-1137, 1989.

Sussman GL, Beezhold DH: Allergy to latex rubber, *Ann Intern Med* 122:43-46, 1995.

Sussman GL, Tarlo S, Dolovich J: The spectrum of IgE-mediated responses to latex, *JAMA* 265:2844-2847, 1991.

Tarlo SM, Sussman G, Contala A, Swanson MC: Control of airborne latex by use of powder-free latex gloves, *J Allergy Clin Immunol* 93:985-989, 1994.

Tarlo SM, Wong L, Roos J et al: Occupational asthma caused by latex in a surgical glove manufacturing plant, *J Allergy Clin Immunol* 85:626-631, 1990.

Taylor J, Evey P, Helm T et al: Contact urticaria and anaphylaxis from latex, *Contact Dermatitis* 23:277-279, 1990.

Turjanmaa K: Incidence of immediate allergy to latex gloves in hospital personnel, *Contact Dermatitis* 17:270-275, 1987.

Turjanmaa K, Laurila K, Mäkinen-Kiljunen S et al: Rubber contact urticaria: allergic properties of 19 brands of latex gloves, *Contact Dermatitis* 19:362-367, 1988a.

Turjanmaa K, Reunala T, Räsänen L: Comparison of diagnostic methods in latex surgical glove contact urticaria, *Contact Dermatitis* 19:241-247, 1988b.

Turjanmaa K, Mäkinen-Kiljunen S, Reunala T et al: Natural rubber latex allergy: the European experience. In Fink J, editor: *Latex allergy: immunology and allergy clinics of North America,* vol 15, Philadelphia, 1995, WB Saunders.

Turjanmaa K, Alenius H, Mäkinen-Kiljunen S et al: Natural rubber allergy. In Kanerva L, Elsner P, Wahlberg JE, Maibach HI, editors: *Handbook of occupational dermatology,* Berlin, 2000, Springer.

Wrangsjö K: Latex allergy in medical, dental, and laboratory personnel: a follow-up study, *Am J Contact Dermat* 5:194-200, 1994.

Yunginger JW, Jones RT, Fransway AF et al: Extractable latex allergens and proteins in disposable medical gloves and other rubber products, *J Allergy Clin Immunol* 93:836-842, 1994.

Carbonless Copy Paper

Carbonless copy paper is a unique recording system that replaced the need for carbon paper. The top sheet is coated on the undersurface with a suspension of microcapsules containing a colorless dye. The underneath sheet is coated on the front with a color developing material. When pressure is applied to the top sheet, the microcapsules are broken and the colorless dye reacts with the color-developing material to result in visualization of the dye. Manufacturers use different solvents, color formers, capsule walls, coreactive surfaces, and paper. Theoretically, any of these substances could cause irritant or allergic skin symptoms.

A common reaction attributed to carbonless copy paper is irritation of the skin and mucous membranes. Symptoms include hoarseness, fatigue, headache, nausea, itching and redness of the skin, and burning of the eyes, nose, mouth, and chest. These symptoms occur predominantly in office workers who handle a lot of carbonless copy paper. The evidence incriminating carbonless copy paper as causing these symptoms was circumstantial until Marks and others (1984) described a 27-year-old woman who had pruritus, eye and throat irritation, hoarseness, shortness of breath, and fatigue within half an hour of exposure to carbonless copy paper. On two separate occasions, when challenged with portions of the paper, contact urticaria and upper airway obstruction developed in this woman. The cutaneous and respiratory symptoms were probably related to prostaglandin release. Investigation of the woman's workplace found 9 of 59 workers with similar symptoms that were related to high exposure to carbonless copy paper. La Marten and others (1988) subsequently described acute systemic reactions to carbonless copy paper that were associated with histamine release. They proved that alkylphenol novolac resin that is present in carbonless copy paper produced contact urticaria and laryngeal edema that could be potentially life-threatening. Hannuksela and Björksten (1989) within a 2-year period saw four female office workers with chronic palmar dermatitis. These workers handled carbonless copy paper for several hours per day. Contact urticaria test results using sheets of the carbonless copy paper were clearly positive: localized wheals and erythema developed. These authors suggested that immediate-type skin reactions appearing as contact urticaria and chronic hand dermatitis may be more common than assumed in office personnel. All four patients were able to continue office work by reducing their contact with carbonless copy paper.

> **Carbonless copy paper has caused contact urticaria, laryngeal edema, and upper airway obstruction in workers who handle this paper.**

However, controlled studies could not prove that carbonless copy paper caused complaints similar to the above mentioned case reports (Jeansson and others, 1984; Murray, 1991). Systematical studies on large groups of humans using repeat insult patch tests showed that carbonless copy paper has produced neither primary skin irritation nor skin sensitization under exaggerated test conditions, demonstrating that neither irritation nor sensitization is expected on contact with carbonless copy paper under normal conditions of manufacture and use (Graves and others, 2000).

BIBLIOGRAPHY

Graves CG, Matanoski GM, Tardiff RG: Carbonless copy paper and workplace safety: a review, *Regul Toxicol Pharmacol* 32:99-117, 2000.

Hannuksela M, Björksten F: Immediate-type dermatitis, contact urticaria, and rhinitis from carbonless copy paper: report of four cases. In Frosch PJ et al, editors: *Current topics in contact dermatitis,* Berlin, 1989, Springer-Verlag.

Jeansson I, Löfström A, Lindblom A: Complaints relating to the handling of carbonless copy paper in Sweden, *Am Ind Hyg Assoc J* 45:B24-B27, 1984.

La Marten FP, Merchant JA, Casale TB: Acute systemic reactions to carbonless copy paper associated with histamine release, *JAMA* 260:242-243, 1988.

Marks JG, Trautlein JJ, Zwillich CW et al: Contact urticaria and airway obstruction from carbonless copy paper, *JAMA* 252:1038-1040, 1984.

Murray R: Health aspects of carbonless copy paper, *Contact Dermatitis* 24:321-333, 1991.

Foods

Foods including dairy products, fruits, grains, nuts, meats, poultry, seafood, and vegetables are among the most common agents that produce immediate contact reactions. Food-related urticarial lesions or flare of dermatitis at the areas of contact have received increasing attention over the last 20 years and have been described, especially in food handlers and housewives. The term *protein contact dermatitis* has been used to describe the chronic hand dermatitis in food handlers that follows allergic contact urticaria from proteinaceous material in foods. Although the skin is relatively impermeable to large macromolecules such as protein allergens, exposure through skin contact can produce both immediate and delayed contact allergy. Atopic or work-related irritant dermatitis causes increased skin permeability and thus plays an important role in the development of contact urticaria. Occupational hand eczema in workers preparing foods was found to be a combination of type 1 and type 4 sensitivities. Hjorth and Roed-Petersen (1976) investigated 33 sandwich makers, kitchen workers, and chefs with hand eczema that was evident in fingertip dermatitis corresponding to the sites of contact with food during its preparation. These workers noticed that within half an hour of handling fish or vegetables, irritation of the hands developed and was followed by redness and vesiculation. Ten of the individuals had positive scratch test reactions only and were determined to have protein contact dermatitis. Fifteen had positive scratch and patch test responses. Six had positive patch test results alone, and two were considered to have irritant contact dermatitis. Application of the incriminated food on healed eczematous skin caused itching, erythema, and in some cases vesiculation within half an hour. Fish and shellfish were the most frequent allergens causing immediate reactions. Onion and garlic were the most common delayed allergens.

A prototype of occupational protein contact dermatitis skin is *baker's eczema*. Many different proteins were identified as allergenic in wheat flour, especially in the water-soluble albumin and globulin fractions. Enzymes and other flour additives are also recognized to be important allergens.

Contact urticaria caused by fruits and vegetables is also a common finding in food industry workers, food handlers, and housewives. Clinical studies suggest that fruit and vegetable allergy is connected with birch pollen allergy. Of 230 patients allergic to birch pollen, 152 (66%) gave a history of immediate reactions provoked by food allergens. Positive scratch-chamber test results with suspected raw fruits and vegetables occurred in 36% of these patients. Apple, carrot, parsnip, and potato elicited the most frequent reactions. The relevance of these positive skin test reactions was found in 80% to 90% of these patients. Radioallergosorbent test studies confirmed a cross-allergy between birch pollen and fruits and vegetables. This suggested that immunologic determinants are shared between pollen and these fruits and vegetables. Birch pollen allergy is associated not only with allergy to fruits and vegetables, but also with allergy to spices, such as paprika, coriander, caraway, cayenne, and mustard.

> **Many foods cause contact urticaria of the hands and oropharynx, particularly fish and shellfish.**

In some individuals with skin contact urticaria that is due to foods, immediate reactions can also occur in the orolaryngeal area that are manifested by itching, tingling, edema of the lips and tongue, and hoarseness or irritation of the throat.

Numerous case reports have described individuals who are sensitive to various foods. This sensitivity may be an underestimated cause of hand dermatitis among housewives. In most cases cooking the food abolishes the type 1 allergic reaction.

BIBLIOGRAPHY

Ale SI, Maibach HI: Occupational contact urticaria. In Kanerva L, Elsner P, Wahlberg JE, Maibach HI, editors: *Handbook of occupational dermatology,* Berlin, 2000, Springer.

Chan EF, Mowad C: Contact dermatitis to foods and spices, *Am J Contact Dermat* 9:71-79, 1998.

Hannuksela M, Lathi A: Immediate reactions to fruits and vegetables, *Contact Dermatitis* 3:70-84, 1977.

Herxheimer H: The skin sensitivity to flour in baker's apprentices, *Lancet* 1:83-84, 1967.

Hjorth N, Roed-Petersen J: Occupational protein contact dermatitis in food handlers, *Contact Dermatitis* 2:28-42, 1976.

Niinimäki A, Hannuksela M, Makinen-Kiljunen S: Skin prick tests and in vitro immunoassays with native spices and spice extracts, *Ann Allergy Asthma Immunol* 75:280-286, 1995.

Tosti A, Fanti PA, Guerra L et al: Morphological and immunohistochemical study of immediate contact dermatitis of the hands due to foods, *Contact Dermatitis* 22:81-85, 1990.

Wuthrich B: Food-induced cutaneous adverse reactions, *Allergy* 53:131-135, 1998.

CHAPTER 17

Contact Dermatitis in Children

The true incidence of childhood allergic contact dermatitis is unknown. In a large population-based study of 1501 eighth-grade students (12 to 16 years old) in Denmark, Mortz and colleagues (2001) reported a point prevalence of contact allergy of 15.2% and a history of present or past contact dermatitis in 7.2% of the children. Girls were twice as likely to have the condition as boys. In a retrospective study of over 4000 visits to a pediatric dermatology clinic in Thailand, 4.9% of the children less than 13 years of age were diagnosed with contact dermatitis (Wisuthsarewong and Viravan, 2000). Still, this type of dermatitis is probably more common than generally recognized. This low index of suspicion coupled with a perception that patch testing of individuals in this age-group is difficult or dangerous has led to infrequent patch testing of children.

There is experimental evidence that children, even newborns, can be sensitized to universal antigens such as *Rhus* species and dinitrochlorobenzene, but at a somewhat lower rate than adults. In a study of 85 asymptomatic normal children below the age of 5 years, patch testing to a standard series of allergens revealed positive patch tests in 24.5% (Bruckner and others, 2000). In contrast, the incidence of response to irritants in childhood appears to decrease with an increase in age between 1 and 7 or 8 years.

In clinical studies the incidence of positive, clinically relevant patch test responses in groups of children who were patch tested has varied from 9% to as high as 70%. This large range is due primarily to the selection of the population to be tested and secondarily to selection of the antigens tested.

One major concern in testing, in view of the increased susceptibility to irritancy in young skin, is that the standard concentrations that are used to test adults will result in irritant or false-positive responses in children. This fear does not appear to be warranted, at least in children older than 3 years of age.

There are technical concerns about testing in young children. Patch testing may mean restriction of activities for a number of days but, since the procedure is painless, most children tolerate it without difficulty. Even infants can be tested when necessary.

One might expect an increase in the incidence of contact sensitivity as an individual ages, simply because the individual is gradually being exposed to a growing number of possible sensitizers. This is in fact borne out by clinical studies. However, some antigens are ubiquitous and occur even in the limited environment of infancy. The most frequent allergens identified as producing positive patch test reactions in groups of children were mercury compounds and nickel. The mercury compounds giving positive results included thimerosal and ethylmecuric chloride. Girls routinely had higher rates of sensitization and were more likely to react to nickel than boys. As in adults, increased nickel sensitivity in females probably relates to ear piercing. In some cultures piercing is frequently done in infancy and childhood. There is a report of a 1-month-old child who was sensitive to nickel (positive test) after ear piercing. Other common sensitizers include rubber components and potassium dichromate causing shoe contact dermatitis; ethylenediamine hydrochloride, neomycin, thimerosal, and benzocaine in topical medicaments; and fragrances and preservatives in cosmetics.

The major difficulty in managing children with allergic contact dermatitis may not be diagnosis, but instruction in allergen avoidance. This may be a particular problem in children who attend school or day-care facilities and in whom the antigen source is not obvious, such as shoes, a medicament, or some household agent. Parents must be given guidance and encouraged to do site visits to identify antigen sources outside the home. Such visits are analogous to the plant visits in occupational dermatitis. Identification of antigen source and instruction in avoidance are even more significant in children if one realizes that antigen avoidance is a lifelong process.

Patch testing of children should be done as outlined for adults. The only limitation may be the surface area of skin that is available for testing. This could limit the number of antigens tested performed at one time. Antigen selection is directed by the history and physical examination, and we recommend always testing with the standard tray.

BIBLIOGRAPHY

Bruckner AL, Weston WL, Morelli JG: Does sensitization to contact allergens begin in infancy? *Pediatrics* 105:e3, 2000.

Cohen PR, Cardullo AC, Ruszkowski AM et al: Allergic contact dermatitis to nickel in children with atopic dermatitis, *Ann Allergy* 65:73-79, 1990.

Fisher AA: Contact leukoderma (vitiligo) hyperpigmentation and discolorations due to contactants. In Fisher AA, editor: *Contact dermatitis,* ed 3, Philadelphia, 1986, Lea & Febiger.

Fisher AA: *Contact dermatitis,* ed 3, Philadelphia, 1986, Lea & Febiger.

Fowler JF: School-days dermatitis, *Am J Contact Dermat* 2:3-4, 1991.

Levy A, Hanau D, Fousserau J: Contact dermatitis in children, *Contact Dermatitis* 6:260-262, 1980.

Mortz CG, Lauritsen JM, Bindslev-Jensen C, Andersen KE: Prevalence of atopic dermatitis, asthma, allergic rhinitis, and hand and contact dermatitis in adolescents: the Odense adolescence cohort study on atopic diseases and dermatitis, *Br J Dermatol* 144:523-532, 2001.

Motolese A, Manzini BM, Donini M: Patch testing in infants, *Am J Contact Dermat* 6:153-156, 1995.

Penny I, Brennestuhl M, Razinskas: Patch testing in children. I. Collective test results, *Contact Dermatitis* 11:201-206, 1984.

Penny I, Brennestuhl M, Razinskas J: Patch testing in children. II. Results and case reports, *Contact Dermatitis* 11:302-310, 1984.

Wantke F, Hemmer W, Jarisch R, Gotz M: Patch test reactions in children, adults and the elderly: a comparative study in patients with suspected allergic contact dermatitis, *Contact Dermatitis* 34:316-319, 1996.

Wisuthsarewong W, Viravan S: Analysis of skin diseases in a referral pediatric dermatology clinic in Thailand, *J Med Assoc Thai* 83:999-1004, 2000.

Index